Explorations in Global Media Ethics

Studies of global media and journalism have repeatedly returned to discussions of ethics. This book highlights the difficulty that journalists encounter when establishing appropriate ethical practices and marks the pressing importance of global media ethics as a subject of current debate. A wide range of contributors – both scholars and practitioners of journalism – identify how changes in journalism practice, developments in new media technologies, legal regulations, and shifting patterns of ownership all play a role in creating ethical tensions for journalists, with some chapters in the book suggesting practical solutions to this pertinent issue. The growing need to faithfully represent other diverse cultural groups is also considered, with certain chapters discussing the impact that human rights, freedom and justice have upon journalistic decision making.

Explorations in Global Media Ethics recognizes that, with the escalation of globalization and a public striving for honest quality media, journalists around the world face an increasing pressure to comply with and simultaneously satisfy diverse ethical practices at both a local and a more global level. The book sympathises with the position of the journalist and calls for greater consideration of his ambiguous role.

This book was originally published as a special issue of *Journalism Studies*.

Muhammad Ayish is currently on leave as a media researcher and consultant in Ottawa, Canada. He holds a doctoral degree in International Communication and Public Diplomacy from the University of Minnesota, Twin Cities, USA (1986). He worked as Dean of the College of Communication at the University of Sharjah (2002–2008). He has authored/co-authored three books on Arab media; the most recent on Arab media industries was published by Polity Press, London. He has had over 60 articles published in international journals on Arab broadcasting, women and media, and political communication.

Shakuntala Rao is a Professor at the State University of New York, USA and has published extensively in Communication and interdisciplinary journals on South Asian journalism postcolonial theory, and media ethics. She received her PhD from the University of Massachusetts, Amherst, USA.

Journalism Studies: Theory and Practice

Series editor: Bob Franklin, Cardiff School of Journalism, Media and Cultural Studies, UK

The journal *Journalism Studies* was established at the turn of the new millennium by Bob Franklin. It was launched in the context of a burgeoning interest in the scholarly study of journalism and an expansive global community of journalism scholars and researchers. The ambition was to provide a forum for the critical discussion and study of journalism as a subject of intellectual inquiry but also an arena of professional practice. Previously, the study of journalism in the UK and much of Europe was a fairly marginal branch of the larger disciplines of media, communication and cultural studies; only a handful of Universities offered degree programmes in the subject. *Journalism Studies* has flourished and succeeded in providing the intended public space for discussion of research on key issues within the field, to the point where in 2007 a sister journal, *Journalism Practice,* was launched to enable an enhanced focus on practice-based issues, as well as foregrounding studies of journalism education, training and professional concerns. Both journals are among the leading ranked journals within the field and publish six issues annually, in electronic and print formats. From the outset, the publication of themed issues has been a commitment for both journals. Their purpose is first, to focus on highly significant or neglected areas of the field; second, to facilitate discussion and analysis of important and topical policy issues; and third, to offer readers an especially high quality and closely focused set of essays, analyses and discussions.

The *Journalism Studies: Theory and Practice* book series draws on a wide range of these themed issues from both journals and thereby extends the critical and public forum provided by them. The Editor of the journals works closely with guest editors to ensure that the books achieve relevance for readers and the highest standards of research rigour and academic excellence. The series makes a significant contribution to the field of journalism studies by inviting distinguished scholars, academics and journalism practitioners to discuss and debate the central concerns within the field. It also reaches a wider readership of scholars, students and practitioners across the social sciences, humanities and communication arts, encouraging them to engage critically with, but also to interrogate, the specialist scholarly studies of journalism which this series provides.

Previously published titles:

Mapping the Magazine
Comparative Studies in Magazine
    Journalism
Edited by Tim Holmes

The Future of Newspapers
Edited by Bob Franklin

Language and Journalism
Edited by John Richardson

The Future of Journalism
Edited by Bob Franklin

New and forthcoming for 2012:

Exploration in Global Media Ethics
*Edited by Muhammad Ayish and
    Shakuntala Rao*

Foreign Correspondence
*Edited by John Maxwell Hamilton and
    Regina G. Lawrence*

How Journalism Uses History
Edited by Martin Conboy

Lifestyle Journalism
Edited by Folker Hanusch

Explorations in Global Media Ethics

Edited by
Muhammad Ayish and Shakuntala Rao

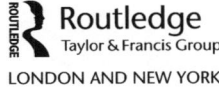

LONDON AND NEW YORK

First published 2012
by Routledge
2 Park Square, Milton Park, Abingdon, Oxon, OX14 4RN

Simultaneously published in the USA and Canada
by Routledge
711 Third Avenue, New York, NY 10017

Routledge is an imprint of the Taylor & Francis Group, an informa business

This book is a reproduction of *Journalism Studies*, volume 12, issue 6. The Publisher requests to those authors who may be citing this book to state, also, the bibliographical details of the special issue on which the book was based.

British Library Cataloguing in Publication Data
A catalogue record for this book is available from the British Library

ISBN13: 978-0-415-62285-1

Typeset in Helvetica
by Taylor & Francis Books

Publisher's Note
The publisher would like to make readers aware that the chapters in this book may be referred to as articles as they are identical to the articles published in the special issue. The publisher accepts responsibility for any inconsistencies that may have arisen in the course of preparing this volume for print.

MIX
Paper from
responsible sources
FSC® C004839
www.fsc.org

Printed and bound in Great Britain by
TJ International Ltd, Padstow, Cornwall

Contents

NOTES ON CONTRIBUTORS

Abeer Al-Najjar holds a PhD in International Journalism from Edinburgh University, UK. Currently she works as an Assistant Professor in Media Studies at the American University of Sharjah, United Arab Emirates. Dr. Al-Najjar has worked in print and broadcast media in Jordan. She has several publications including a book titled *Conflict Over Jerusalem: covering the Palestinian-Israeli conflict in the British press* (2009). She has also published journal articles and book chapters and held presentations specifically on the interconnectivity of media, politics and religion, social media and social movements, a comparative study of Al-Jazeera Arabic and Al-Jazeera English, social media, the Gaza War, and the Palestinian Identity, and the content and ideology in news media. Her research focuses on Arab media, social media and popular culture. Al-Najjar is a member of the editorial board of the Palgrave Macmillan Series in Global Public Diplomacy.

Muhammad Ayish is currently on leave as a media researcher and consultant in Ottawa, Canada. He holds a doctoral degree in International Communication and Public Diplomacy from the University of Minnesota, Twin Cities, USA (1986). He worked as Dean of the College of Communication at the University of Sharjah (2002–2008). He has authored/co-authored three books on Arab media; the most recent on Arab media industries was published by Polity Press, London. He has had over 60 articles published in international journals on Arab broadcasting, women and media, and political communication.

Abderrahmane Azzi is currently a Professor at the University of Sharjah, United Arab Emirates. Dr. Azzi holds a PhD in the Sociology of Mass Communication (1985) from North Texas State University, USA. Dr. Azzi has almost 30 years experience of teaching and research. He has taught at NTSU, the University of Algiers, the International Islamic University Malaysia, King Saud University and the United Arab Emirates University. He has published and co-authored numerous books and published more than 40 studies in many academic journals in Arabic and English. His research and interests are in the field of moral communication.

Clifford G. Christians is a Research Professor of Communications, Professor of Journalism, and Professor of Media Studies Emeritus at the University of Illinois-Urbana, USA. He served as Director of the Institute of Communications Research from 1987 to 2001 and 2007 to 2009. He is the author or co-author of such books as *Media Ethics: cases and moral reasoning*, *Jacques Ellul: interpretive essays*, *Good News: social ethics, press, communication ethics and universal values*, *Moral Engagement in Public Life: theorists for contemporary ethics*, *Normative Theories of the Media*, *Key Concepts in Critical Cultural*

Studies, *Handbook of Mass Media Ethics*, and *Ethical Communication: five moral stances in human dialogue.*

James Piecowye earned his PhD in Communication from the University of Montreal, Canada. Piecowye began teaching at Zayed University in Dubai in 2000 and became a talk show host on Dubai Eye radio in 2006. He has a keen interest in Media Literacy and is working on the creation of the Gulf Media Literacy Initiative to serve private and public education environments in the United Arab Emirates.

Shakuntala Rao received her PhD from the University of Massachusetts, Amherst, USA. She is a Professor at the State University of New York, Plattsburgh, USA and has published extensively in Communication and interdisciplinary journals on South Asian journalism postcolonial theory, and media ethics. She has been a senior Fulbright scholar to India and has been Visiting Professor at universities in Pakistan and Sri Lanka.

Stephen J. A. Ward is the James E. Burgess Professor of Journalism Ethics in the School of Journalism and Mass Communication at the University of Wisconsin-Madison, USA. He is the author of *The Invention of Journalism Ethics: the path to objectivity and beyond* (2005), *Global Journalism Ethics* (2010) and co-editor of *Media Ethics Beyond Borders: a global perspective* (2009). Ward is also Associate Editor of the *Journal of Mass Media Ethics*. He was a reporter, war correspondent, and newsroom manager for 14 years. He covered conflicts in Yugoslavia, Bosnia and Northern Ireland and was the British Columbia bureau chief for the Canadian press news agency in Vancouver.

Herman Wasserman is the Deputy Head of the School of Journalism and Media Studies, Rhodes University, South Africa. He worked previously as a journalist for the Cape Town-based daily, *Die Burger*. He is the Editor of *Ecquid Novi: African Journal for Journalism Research*. He is the author of *Tabloid Journalism in South Africa* and co-editor of *Shifting Selves: post-apartheid essays on mass media, culture and identity* (with Sean Jacobs) and *Media Ethics Beyond Borders: a global perspective* (with Stephen J. A. Ward).

Lee Wilkins is Curator's Teaching Professor at the School of Journalism, University of Missouri, USA. She is co-author of the best-selling college ethics text, *Media Ethics: issues and cases* and the Editor of the leading academic journal on media ethics, the *Journal of Mass Media Ethics*. Her co-edited book with Clifford G. Christians, *Handbook of Mass Media Ethics*, was named the best edited book of 2009 by the ethics division of the National Communication Association. Prior to her academic appointments, Wilkins served as a newspaper editor and reporter in Colorado, Oregon and Michigan.

PREFACE

This special issue of *Journalism Studies* reflects the perennial preoccupation of scholars of journalism studies with ethical questions and debates. Changes in journalism practice, developments in new media technologies, as well as shifting patterns of ownership, regulation and organisation of the media and journalism industries in the age of global media, make these "preoccupations" more urgent and pertinent than ever. As the Guest Editors of this collection of papers argue, "audiences around the world continue to desire quality journalism, and thinking through an ethics of journalism and media that reflects changes in the media, marketplace, and political landscapes as well as in contemporary philosophy becomes an urgent task".

The articles published in this issue of *Journalism Studies* by both scholars and practitioners of journalism, began life as papers presented to the Global Media Ethics Roundtable organised at Zayed University on 22–24 March 2010, in Dubai, United Arab Emirates. I am grateful to Guest Editors Muhammad Ayish and Shakuntala Rao for their efforts in convening such a distinguished group of scholarly contributors whose thought-provoking studies make a substantial contribution to our understanding of global media and journalism ethics.

I would also like to express my gratitude to John C. Merrill, Professor Emeritus at Missouri University and Linda Steiner, Professor and Director of Research and Doctoral Studies at the Philip Merrill College of Journalism, University of Maryland, for reading and offering helpful comments on all of the articles published here.

BOB FRANKLIN
Editor

INTRODUCTION
Explorations in global media ethics

Muhammad Ayish and **Shakuntala Rao**

Studies of global media and journalism have repeatedly returned to discussions of ethics. Philosophical models of interpretation have consistently informed analyses and cognizance of the fast changing media landscape. In the era of globalization and the "post-postmodernization" of the world as marked by the birth of new nations, decolonization, the end of Soviet hegemony, and the rising consciousness of democracy, we become increasingly obligated to pay attention to the multi-layered exploitations of development in the form of migrant labor, sex industries, and sweat shops. The question posed by Wasserman (2008, p. 92), "Is it possible to agree on ethical conduct for journalists around the globe?" has become an urgent one. New media technologies, as well as the processes of media liberalization, deregulation, and privatization across national boundaries, have altered journalism as a profession. While journalism has stayed firmly anchored in the local, often adapting, appropriating, and localizing global practices and technologies, a vision for global journalism ethics remains only partially articulated. Study after study shows that audiences around the world continue to desire quality journalism, and thinking through an ethics of journalism and media that reflects changes in the media, marketplace, and political landscapes as well as in contemporary philosophy becomes an urgent task. "If news media are to be guided by universal ethics, then journalists need to reconceive their role as major players in cross-cultural discourse", write Christians et al., "the first step is to reconsider journalists as active inquirers who should seek to provide nuanced and informed interpretations of their world, while being fully aware of the difficulties of representing others" (2008, p. 139). Journalists and media professionals require not only an understanding of the ongoing philosophical debate about the accommodation of otherness, but should work with a framework of concrete universals, one which *transforms* universalism, rather than abandoning it, while attempting to redress the coercive, manipulative, and exclusionary application of the "universal".

The coeval perturbations of the theory revolution and canonical revisionism of the 1970s, felt first and most profoundly in the disciplines of literature, philosophy, and anthropology, challenged and transformed ethical theory in most professions. Ethics talk has been re-legitimized during the past two decades by currents within "high theory": by Foucault's reevaluation of the category of the self, conceiving of care as an ethical project among Feminist writers, and Derrida's desconstructive critical practice as itself an ethics. Philosophers, such as Carey, Couldry, and Nussbaum have themselves turned to media and journalism to examine and express ethical reflection. These theoretical debates penetrated studies of media and journalism practices as the Birmingham Center for Contemporary Cultural Studies, and by Christians and his colleagues, integrated insights from Communitarianism into studies of media and journalism.

Contemporary debates on media and journalism ethics appear to come to an impasse in the confrontation between two positions, the one (identity politics) vying to assert absolute difference between culturally constituted human beings, and the other (neo-Kantian proceduralism) arguing for sameness based in the common "humanity" of all human beings. While the claimants for the "sameness" of all human beings accuse the proponents of difference of promoting radical relativism, the proponents of acknowledging and accepting difference accuse the universalists of trying to impose (usually Western) values onto (sometimes colonized) people. Instead of remaining in such a polarized, and paralyzed, argument, we can start with a study of current philosophical debates around ethics which would not only show that we are intellectually current, responsible, and rigorous, but also will give us hope about creating a revitalized, effective, and future-oriented global media ethics. And if we are to proceed with some degree of intellectual possibilities (and hope), studies of media and journalism should confront such questions without lapsing into metaphysics, total undecidability, or simply, political disaffectedness. We begin by invoking Appiah's (2006, p. 118) simple question, "Why the need to consider the ethics of the other?"

At the center of negotiating the universal–particular, self–other debates in ethics has been the difficult concept of culture (media often has become the conduit through which culture is defined, captured, or critiqued), encoded in the language of cultural rights and choices. Universal ethics should be rejected, one could thus argue, because it infringes on the terrain of "my" culture's ethics. Many theorists have argued that culture is constituted by encounters with the other and that culture and identity are hybrid and dynamic (see Ayish and Azzi's articles in this issue). Geertz and others have tried to challenge the idea of culture-as-self-containedness by taking on the responsibility of engaging with "strangeness" as constitutive of the very moment of cultural identification and ethical enunciation. Geertz asks us "to refocus our attention and make us visible to ourselves by representing us and everyone else as cast into the midst of a world full of irremovable strangeness we can't keep clear of" (1986, p. 121). Encounters with such cultural strangeness cannot be regulated in a binary representation of cultural difference as "us-versus-them." The problem is not, Geertz warns "the distant tribe enfolded upon itself in coherent difference" but a disjunctive, anxious terrain of "sudden faults and dangerous passages" that produce moral asymmetries within the boundary of a "we" (1986, p. 121). The making of the "we", Geertz argues, is not limited to the West though it has been most highlighted in the post-Enlightenment citizen as a political subject (the conflation of the outsider in Euroamerican sense with the global outsider should be avoided, the "we" here could constitute identity as much for Algerians in France as for Tibetans in China and South Asian migrants in the Middle East). Such strangeness is oblique and shaded, less easily set off as anomalous as it is "scrambled together in ill-defined expanses, social spaces whose edges are unfixed, irregular, and difficult to locate" (Geertz, 1986, p. 121). For Bhabha, culture is highly productive and he proposes "ethos and poetics of identification" which represents the process through which international relations *in between* class, gender, generation, race, religion, or region are articulated as hybrid identifications and that identities are produced in the "intersective or interstital cultural processes" rather than in any claim of originary self-definition with free access to "moral or mimetic measure of cultural knowledge" (2000, p. 188). If culture is a regulator to how someone knows and taxonomies of culture are possible and useful, while recognizing that any culture at work is also, as Spivak notes, a play of differences from these taxonomies. "Culture alive is always on the run" Spivak writes, "always changeful" (2008, p. 357), the fear is until culture, in broad strokes, starts "speaking in the name of political, ethical, and other narratives" (p. 359).

Ethicists are starting to move away, in as much practice of ethics for media and journalism as in the theory of media and journalism ethics, from an articulation that cultural difference can only be achieved by acknowledging values within any one cultural system, to a wider position that judgments across cultures (universal) can be linked to and be tolerant of ontological rights of self-representation (particular). Appiah, Taylor, Foucault, and others, have thought about how pluralist democracies can ensure the coexistence of a potentially infinite array of diverse ethical systems and approaches. While the solutions of interlocutors in these discussions vary, to the point of seeming irreconcilable, all appear animated by a genuine commitment to an ethos of "recognition of difference" (Appiah, 2006, p. 118). Journalism and media ethicists could also problematize universalism, while taking seriously the various philosophies and histories of others. Like the philosophers working on the question of ethics and the other, we can try to think through a series of questions: "How can we combine a commitment to the universal recognition of others with respect for the concrete particularism, difference, or asymmetry of others?"; "How can we dispel the generalized figment of the "generalized other" that dominates versions of the universal in order to acknowledge particularlized others?"; "How can we avoid reifying the otherness of the other so as to turn him or her into an abstract alterity?"; and, most crucially, "How can we try to redress the violence enacted by hegemonic discourses that silence or slight the subaltern other?" Studies of global media and journalism should confront such questions. The essays in this issue, when read collectively, not only present a mix of theoretical frameworks and case-studies but seek connections between global media ethics and regional approaches, theories, and professional practices. For journalists and media practitioners, the efforts at seeking "human-centered global proto-norms" (Christians et al., 2008), we believe, require such connections.

Grappling with changes in technology, globalization and ethical theory during the past decade, journalism and media professionals have made various efforts to develop a philosophically rigorous and epistemologically sound ethics for the global media (Brislin, 2004; Christians and Traber, 1997; Couldry, 2006; Merrill, 2002; Silverstone, 2007; Ward, 2010). In one attempt to formulate global media ethics, the *Journal of Mass Media Ethics* published a special issue titled, "Search for a Global Media Ethics" (2003). In this issue, Callahan writes that the profession's global scope and transnational media provokes the question of whether there can be "universal ethical standards for journalism to meet the challenges of globalization" (Callahan, 2003, p. 3). Similarly, Ward (2005, p. 4) states that a global media ethics would imply that responsibility "would be owed to an audience scattered across the world", given the increasingly global reach of media corporations facilitated through new technologies. Christians and Nordenstreng (2004) have proposed a theoretical formulation which re-examines the search for global media ethics, and proposes the social responsibility theory as a possibility for the press to adopt internationally. They offer the possibility of establishing several universal principles which they ground in "a morality rooted in animate nature" (2004, p. 20). Stating that "global social responsibility needs an ethical basis commensurate in scope, that is, universal ethical principles rather than the parochial moral guidelines represented by codes", Christians and Nordenstreng list respect for human dignity based on sacredness of human life, truth, and non-violence as three universal principles (2004, p. 20). Ward and Wasserman, in the introduction of their book *Media Ethics Beyond Borders: a global perspective*, one of the first comprehensive anthologies on global media ethics, write,

"A global-minded media is of significant value because biased and parochial media can wreak havoc in a tightly linked global world. By the same token, media that claim to be 'global' yet fail to acknowledge the ways in which their ethical perspectives are influenced by their own cultural, historical or political positioning, will be unable to help us make sense of the world in which we live" (2008, p. 1). Ethicists, journalists, and scholars alike agree that any invention, evolution, or construction of global media and journalism ethics should be highly nuanced both in its epistemological approaches and in practical applications.

Christians et al. (2008), in their essay on global media ethics, propose a cross-disciplinary theoretical perspective. The essay does not presume to provide conclusive answers to theoretical questions about the relationship between the self and the other, the local and the global, or the universal and the particular, but puts forward an argument about ways in which current disagreements about the nature, possibility, and desirability of a global media ethics could be addressed. "Progress in developing a global media ethics is stymied by a number of wide-spread beliefs and presumptions," write Christians et al. The authors contend that "One issue is whether there *are* universal values in media ethics." Their answer is a qualified "yes"; they write:

> It appears there are universals. Even a cursory survey of many codes of journalism ethics would find agreement, at least on a denotative level, on such values as reporting the truth, freedom, and independence, minimizing harm, and accountability. Yet, a survey would also find differences. Some media cultures emphasize more strongly than others such values as the promotion of social solidarity, not offending religious beliefs and not weakening public support for the military. Even where media systems agree on a value, such as "freedom of press" or "social responsibility", they may interpret and apply such principles in different ways. (Christians et al., 2008, p. 138)

In opening up these tensions, the authors describe several theoretical positions which might coalesce to form our current understanding of global media ethics. In their attempts to avoid errors of the past, Christians et al. propose an outline of a theory of ethics consisting of levels: "the levels of presuppositions, principles, and precepts" (2008, p. 140), that interact dynamically in experience. Rooted in a holistic conception of theory where basic values and ideas emerge from a "common humanness in concrete contexts", Christians et al. see such values as "context-influenced articulations of deep aspects of being human" (2008, p. 139). The most deeply embedded disagreements between factions (agnostic, antifoundationalist, poststructuralist, accounts of pluralism and multiculturalism), the authors argue, should not necessarily detract from the circumstances that they also come together at notable junctures and that most theories of ethics usually subscribe to a modicum of universalization and to some universal extension of nonviolence and sacredness of human life. The authors juxtapose their claim of "humanness" as universal with a critique of past ethicists who did not fully articulate their own theoretical location as imperialist or as historically, culturally, and politically positioned. Christians et al. hope that the global and local can engage in a reflexive, relational, and critical dialectic that could contribute to an extended discussion of ethics for the global media.

Given such contentiousness debates and new ideas in the history of media and journalism debates, the three-day Global Media Ethics Roundtable organized at Zayed University on March 22–24, 2010, in Dubai, United Arab Emirates, gave scholars and practitioners a chance to discuss such debates. The essays in this special issue were presented at the Roundtable. While four of the nine articles at the Roundtable addressed media in the Middle East, the participants consciously tried to move away from the usual diagnosis of Middle Eastern media (as well as of the societies from which such media emerge) as non-plural and parochial and, therefore, as needing intervention from Western journalists and ethicists. These articles were penned much earlier to the citizens' revolutions we have witnessed in some of the countries in the Middle East and the significant role media has played in these revolutions. While such changes could not have been predicted a year earlier, essays in this issue challenge the model of the "clash of civilizations" rhetoric and the subsequent defeat of any composite idea of multi-ethics in journalism and media practices and policies. The conference took place in Dubai, a city which has emerged as a major hub for global media, with a large number of regional and international satellite television news and entertainment networks and because the influx of new media has also radicalized rhetoric, leading some scholars to argue that new media is incompatible with the region's social and cultural traditions and indigenous value systems (Azzi and Meshmeshi, 2010).

While some critics in the region have viewed state-controlled media as part of socially and politically-conscious and benevolent governments, some have interpreted private media, especially satellite television and websites, with their commercial and Western-style formats, as the least committed to regional and local ethical values. Amin (2008), for instance, accuses new media as providing highly sensationalized content, and thus breaching the "standards of public morality", often only to attract more audiences for advertisers. In 2003, for instance, angry demonstrators in Bahrain took to the streets to protest the filming and broadcast of *Big Brother* (renamed in Arabic as *al-Ra'is* or *The Boss*), a reality TV show in which 12 unmarried young men and women are video-taped living under the same roof. The broadcast of *al-Ra'is* was subsequently cancelled. The most recent example of an offensive broadcast featured a Saudi man who bragged of his sexual escapades on a talk-show on Lebanese TV. In response to a petition from thousands of angry protestors, the man was tried in a Saudi court, received lashings, and a long prison sentence.

Increased exposure to Western media content and formats has generated interest in, and concern about, the ethical standards of those media. In tandem with protests about the content of new media, the emergence of satellite news channels like Al Jazeera and Al Arabiya has also posed questions about the implications of applying Western-style journalism ethics in an Arab region marked by state-control of information and cultural conservatism. Such wariness accompanies, and arises out of, raised awareness among media practitioners, journalists, policy makers, and the general public about the need for professional standards in addressing ethical issues. In recent years, journalists, media owners, and policy mavens in the Middle East have begun to recognize that global media does not always or necessarily subvert and erase indigenous (Arab) values. These changes in perceptions of the local/regional versus global/Western ethical divide have inspired some Middle Eastern professionals to try to self-regulate by combining global and local ethical perspectives. While it had been almost impossible, in the past, to discuss media and journalism ethics beyond the cultural and social parameters of Arab–Islamic values and norms, it has become increasingly acceptable to address ethical issues in a "synthesist fashion": one which combines regional and Western media ethics (Ayish, 2008, p. 12).

While Middle Eastern media and journalism ethics codes vary in content, they commonly emphasize freedom, responsibility, privacy, fairness, objectivity, and access to information. The code of ethics developed by the Qatar-based Al Jazeera Satellite Channel (JSC), for example, highlights the hybridity of these codes. The JSC code of ethics states that Al Jazeera "adheres to the journalistic values of honesty, courage, fairness, balance, independence, credibility and diversity, giving no priority to commercial or political considerations over professional ones" (Al Jazeera, 2008). It also states that "the broadcaster will endeavor to get to the truth and declare it in our dispatches, programs and news bulletins unequivocally in a manner which leaves no doubt about its validity and accuracy" (Al Jazeera, 2008). Recent codes of ethics developed in the Middle East have begun to incorporate ethical concepts, such as freedom, balance, and independence, often associated with Western journalism. It is likely that this trend will continue as more media channels, like Al Jazeera, which are based in the Middle East but have global ambitions, emerge and seek global audiences by adopting global ethical standards, and/or by adapting them to local contexts using both local and global ethical standards.

As these examples from the Middle East have shown, ethical universals for the global media continue to be existentially impoverished and need the "thickness of language" (Clifford Christians, personal communcation, 2010) to make them practically relevant and theoretically viable. The explorations in this issue undertakes into the analogues and constituents of global media and journalism ethics: freedom, democracy, patriotism, responsibility, localization, and regionalism addressed from a variety of perspectives. This collective endeavor, the work of many hands, was needed to chart such an intellectual path.

In the first essay of the issue, Christians gives us a philosophy of technology that helps construct ethical universals during an era of globalization. Christians' humanocentric perspective on technology critiques the prevailing view of technology as neutral, and urges journalists and media scholars to consider a human-centered theory of technology. It advocates for accommodating alternative technologies in universal theory and demonstrates the need for transforming values through education, particularly those interested in journalism and media education. Christians hopes that journalists and media scholars construct human-centered global proto-norms in order to question the basic tenets which guide current technocentric societies.

Ward, in his essay, proposes that we reconceive journalism ethics around the idea of ethical flourishing as one interpretation of the human good. Ethical flourishing expresses the impulse of the ethics of cosmopolitanism, which asserts the equal value and dignity of all, as members of a common humanity. Ward suggests we take the aim of ethical flourishing to be global ethical flourishing. To work towards the ethical flourishing of a global community is to promote a cosmopolitanism that emphasizes universal principles of human rights, freedom, and justice. Ward urges journalists and educators to emphasize the representation of others as those others see themselves, since misrepresentation can spark wars, demean already marginalized cultures, and support unjust social structures. Such issues of representing the other's perspective go beyond issues of factual accuracy and fairness, Ward agues, and require journalists to have a deeper cultural knowledge and a deeper appreciation of how language can distort the other.

According to Al-Najjar, in Arab journalism, tensions between professional obliga-tions and patriotism militate against the development of sound ethical standards and any type of global journalism. In her essay, Al-Najjar notes that Arab journalists have to grapple with the double challenge of conforming to government-influenced media practices which emphasize patriotism while working according to Western-style journalism codes that do not address the region's issues. She observes that, especially in times of conflict, Arab journalists are expected by their national governments and audiences to act patriotically while being criticized by international journalism communities for failing to apply ethical journalistic standards of impartiality and objectivity.

In articulating the "ethics of the other" (the West's other), Azzi's essay provides an ethical framework for journalists and media ethics scholars based on reading of the Quran by the eighteenth-century Turkish philosopher, Al Nursi Badi'uzzaman Said. Azzi argues that Al Nursi's work takes a macro-level perspective from Quran which postulates that everything that exists in the Universe is a reflection of one or more of God's attributes (known as the 99 plus in Islam), and he applies this idea to everyday ethical decision making. By providing a normative framework, derived from al Nursi's Sufism, Azzi suggests that journalists, especially in the Middle East, consider six of Al Nursi's interpretation of God's attributes and help them guide in their day-to-day workings.

Ayish, Rao, and Wasserman's essays discuss the intersections of the global and local in three different regional settings: the Middle East, Africa, and South Asia. Because these regions are emerging in importance in the geopolitical future of the world, and because local journalists and media professionals are increasingly scrutinized both in local and Western ethical terms, these essays examine the syntheses of, tensions between, and reciprocal transformations of local and global ethical values. They argue that converging values represent universal proto-norms that are shared by human beings across cultures while diverging values suggest cultural peculiarities of the region. Ayish's essay studies the responses of college students, in Sharjah, United Arab Emirates, to reality television in the region. He concludes that Arab publics' response to both globalized and localized media do not carry clear-cut demarcation between what is to be perceived as ethically good or ethically bad. Results from his interview demonstrate clear preferences for a "glocalized" media ethics rooted in synthesized indigenous and universal values.

Rao argues that studies of media ethics and practices of journalists should research the reciprocity and mutual adaptations of ethical values within regions of/across the borders of nation-states. Studying regional identities and regional media complicates traditional understandings of the "ethics of the other". Rao's article explores critical regionalism, as defined in the works of Gayatri Chakravorty Spivak, as a way to understand and expand the concept of "local" in global media ethics. By using examples of South Asian media—in India and Nepal—the essay concludes that the epistemic inclusion of integrating critical regionalism, contextualized within the broader disciplinary position of Postcolonial theory, into our ethical theory and practice can help us understand the complicated nexus of media ethics, localization, and identity politics.

Wasserman's paper critiques the notions of social responsibility and freedom as normative foundations for global media ethics, by pointing at the conflicting interpreta-tions of these terms and the tensions between them, with examples from journalism practices in Africa. In his interviews with South African and Namibian journalists he finds that journalists position themselves in ethical frameworks ranging from the developmental and indigenization framework to the freedom and social responsibility model. This essay suggests that normative frameworks of journalism ethics are still being contested and negotiated in Africa. It is, therefore, impossible to speak of African, regional, or local ethics except in preliminary terms. Wasserman concludes that comparable historical and contemporary political, social, and cultural factors impact the negotiation of ethical frameworks and that these negotiations are also embedded in wider cultural flows between Africa and the rest of the world: one which problematizes any simple or monolithic understanding of African ethics or journalism ethics in Africa.

For Wilkins, the quest to mark clear boundaries between freedom and individual responsibility should account for "moral reasoning" in ethical decision making. In her essay, she explores the connection between emotions, bounded rationality, and professional ethical decision making, specifically journalistic negotiation between freedom and responsibility. She argues that, based on the findings of neuroscience coupled with feminist ethics, and the concept of proto-norms as outlined by Christians, journalists' moral sentiments regarding these core concepts are linked to the development of a moral imagination that seeks both professionally sound and morally creative alternatives to difficult ethical choices. Wilkins uses a case study of a Cambodian documentary film maker to illustrate the ways emotions and reason converge to define ethical decision making in media work.

Piecowye, a radio talk-show host in Dubai, gives a brief case-study which addresses the difficulty of negotiating global and local ethics. Piecowye describes how he handled a culturally sensitive issue on a live show, *Nightline*, aired on a Dubai-based English-language radio station, Dubai Eye 103.8 FM. On the air, Piecowye discussed the arrest by Dubai police of a British couple who were kissing in public. The case-study shows that local cultural codes of conduct and legal regulations shape ethical decision making among foreign-language radio broadcasters in the United Arab Emirates, despite their attempts to enact global journalistic ethics. Piecowye argues that, while hybridization of culture and media practices increases, major ethical decisions continue to be influenced in the United Arab Emirates, not only by Western theories of press freedom and responsibilities, but, sometimes more strongly, by local ethics codes, laws, and fear of punishment.

ACKNOWLEDGEMENTS

We would like to acknowledge the people who made this special issue possible. We thank Cliord Christians for his unwavering leadership in this project. Both his intellectual and time commitments have impelled many of the achievements of Global Media Ethics Roundtables. We thank the editor of *Journalism Studies*, Bob Franklin, for his support in giving these papers a published home. Thanks also to the Dean of the College of Communication and Media Sciences at Zayed University, Marilyn Roberts, for providing the academic space and an open and inclusive environment for the meeting and discussions. We gratefully acknowledge the work of the organizing committee at Zayed University and, in particular, the tireless eorts of James Piecowye and Andrea Juhasz.

REFERENCES

AL JAZEERA (2008) "Code of Ethics", http://english.aljazeera.net/aboutus/2006/11/2008525185733692771. html, accessed 8 October 2010.

AMIN, HUSSEIN (2008) "The Arab States Charter for Satellite Television: a quest regulation", *Arab Media & Society*, http://www.arabmediasociety.com/?article =649, accessed 10 October 2010.

APPIAH, ANTHONY (2006) *Cosmopolitanism: ethics in the world of strangers*, New York: W. W. Norton.

AYISH, MUHAMMAD (2008) *The New Arab Public Sphere*, Berlin: Frank & Timme.

AZZI, ABDUL RAHMAN and MESHMESHI, MAMDOUH (Eds) (2010) *Arab Satellite Channels and Cultural Identity: vision for media in the 21st century*, Sharjah, UAE: University of Sharjah Publishers.

BHABHA, HOMI (2000) "On Cultural Choice", in: Marjorie Garber, Beatrice Hanssen and Rebecca Walkowitz (Eds), *The Turn to Ethics*, New York: Routledge, pp. 181–200.

BRISLIN, TOM (2004) "Empowerment as a Universal Ethic in Global Journalism", *Journal of Mass Media Ethics* 19(2), pp. 130–7.

CALLAHAN, SIDNEY (2003) "New Challenges of Globalization for Journalism", *Journal of Mass Media Ethics* 18(1), pp. 3–15.

CHRISTIANS, CLIFFORD and NORDENSTRENG, KAARLE (2004) "Social Responsibility Worldwide", *Journal of Mass Media Ethics* 19(1), pp. 3–28.

CHRISTIANS, CLIFFORD and TRABER, MICHAEL (Eds) (1997) *Communication Ethics and Universal Values*, Thousand Oaks, CA: Sage.

CHRISTIANS, CLIFFORD, RAO, SHAKUNTALA, WARD, STEPHEN J. A. and WASSERMAN, HERMAN (2008) "Toward a Global Media Ethics: theoretical perspectives", *Ecquid Novi: African Journalism Studies* 29(2), pp. 135–72.

COULDRY, NICK (2006) *Listening Beyond the Echoes: media, ethics and agency in an uncertain world*, Boulder, CO: Paradigm Publishers.

GEERTZ, CLIFFORD (1986) "The Uses of Diversity and the Future of Ethnocentrism", *Michigan Quarterly Review* 25(1), pp. 105–23.

MERRILL, JOHN (2002) "Chaos and Order: sacrificing the individual for the sake of social harmony", in: Atkins Joseph (Ed.), *The Mission: journalism, ethics and the world*, Ames: Iowa State University Press, pp. 17–36.

SILVERSTONE, ROGER (2007) *Media and Morality: on the rise of the mediapolis*, New York: Polity Press.

SPIVAK, GAYATRI CHAKRAVORTY (2008) *Other Asias*, Malden, MA: Blackwell Publishing.

WARD, STEPHEN J. A. (2005) "Philosophical Foundations for Global Journalism Ethics", *Journal of Mass Media Ethics* 20(1), pp. 3–21.

WARD, STEPHEN J. A. (2010) *Global Journalism Ethics*, Montreal: McGill University Press.

WARD, STEPHEN J. A. and WASSERMAN, HERMAN (2008) "Introduction", in: Stephen J. A. Ward and Herman Wasserman (Eds), *Media Ethics Beyond Borders: a global perspective*, New York: Routledge, pp. 1–4.

WASSERMAN, HERMAN (2008) "Global Journalism Ethics", in: Arnold DeBeer and John Merrill (Eds), *Global Journalism: topical issues and media systems*, New York: Allyn and Bacon, pp. 85–95.

THE PHILOSOPHY OF TECHNOLOGY
Globalization and ethical universals

Clifford G. Christians

The philosophy of technology has a substantive role in constructing ethical universals during an era of globalization. It makes two major contributions to a new generation of media ethics: a critique of the prevailing view of technology as neutral and a human-centered theory of technology. Three applications are pertinent: (1) it prevents us from universals in the Enlightenment tradition; (2) it advocates including alternative technologies in universal theory; and (3) it demonstrates the need for transforming values through education.

The arc of the moral universe is long, but it bends toward justice. (Martin Luther King, Jr.)

Introduction

While we work together on a global media ethics, the concept of globalization is in crisis intellectually and practically. It is now obvious that the idea has been co-opted by the industrial world in terms of marketplace economics. And there is a global meltdown sociologically: the range between rich and poor is higher than ever; the growth of sectarianism and fundamentalism is making democracy nearly impossible; the inequalities of ethnicity, gender, immigration are ferocious; education is cut back while consumerism prospers (Commers et al., 2008). Political economy and cultural studies give us important perspectives, but the philosophy of technology also has a strategic role to play in coming to grips with the issues of globalization. In fact, it offers a substantive framework for constructing a new generation of ethical proto-norms. Rather than the Western rationalist model where universals are categorical, abstract, and imperialistic, the new model is multicultural and gender inclusive. It is multilayered and complex, rather than the single strand principle of the Enlightenment.

While the philosophy of technology gives us a deep reading of the global technological phenomenon, it does not provide a smooth pathway for media ethics. Any credible version of ethical universals requires at least minimal agreement on freedom and responsibility and their relationship. The philosophy of technology considers both to be problematic concepts in highly technological regimes, that is, in both industrial nations and in professions such as journalism that are technologically advanced. Instead of freedom, citizens of and members in those regimes follow technological necessity; instead of ends and responsibility they are driven by means and amorality. Though complicating our forward movement conceptually, the philosophy of technology insures that we make a radical break with conventional thinking on media technology and that we confront the right issues in media ethics.

I am not presenting the traditional dichotomy between the developing and industrial world. The philosophy of technology does not focus on modernization theory, with its trickle-down emphasis on the diffusion of tools. It thinks instead in terms of technological regimes. Some such regimes are geographical: Dubai, world-class high-tech and high-finance innovator; Finland, the largest concentration of Web units in the world; Singapore, an Internet island where every home, office and school is linked to an ultra-fast, multimedia network. Other technological regimes are regional or particular: Silicon Valley, USA, with 5000 communications and cyber companies; ZhongGuanCun, Beijing's international home for ICT entrepreneurs; Rupert Murdoch's News Corporation, with 64,000 employees in news, advertising, entertainment, and media production; Tecnológico de Monterrey, Mexico, specializing in social networking technologies and business incubator models for the knowledge-economy. And some professions are high-technology regimes also: medicine, the military, and international finance, for example. Journalism, advertising, public relations, and entertainment have depended on sophisticated technology since the days of radio and television; digitalization has put media industries on a new order of magnitude.

Instrumentalism

The first major contribution of the philosophy of technology is its critique of the prevailing view in technological regimes. Technology is presumed to be neutral, that is, technology seen in mechanistic terms as tools and products. Technologies are not value-laden but achievements of engineering. If television is excessively violent, we should not blame those who designed and manufactured them. Consumers use bad judgment. If a computer database controls both the Burj Khalifa tower and communications within al Qaeda, technology *per se* is not the issue, but the uses to which we put it.

Although exploding communications technology is increasingly at the forefront of our work on media ethics, it is not the crisis by itself. Instead of glib references to information technology and presuming the technological imperative, media systems must be embedded in their institutional, historical, and sociocultural infrastructure. Ongoing work in the philosophy of technology is indispensable for this substantive task. Since technologies are not neutral but value-laden, intellectual work on the character of media technology as a whole is necessary for the long term.

For the philosophy of technology, the first issue is instrumentalism. The prevailing worldview in industrial societies is instrumentalism—the view, inherited from Aristotle, that technology is neutral and unfolds out of its own character. Technology itself does not condition our humanness. The reverse is true; humans control technology as their purpose and needs require it. In our commonplaces, technologies are seen in mechanistic terms as instruments of engineering apart from values. If the cancer rate goes up from pesticides and if television advertising is exploitative, we should not blame those who designed and manufactured the tools. Politicians and consumers use bad judgment. Technological products are independent, we conclude; they can be used to support completely different cultures and lifestyles (Pacey, 1996). Websites can give us the lives and history of heroes or the hate speech of a fundamentalist sect. Airplanes drop bombs or carry emergency aid to Haiti. Online games can be pornographic or educational. Technology is subordinate to practical wisdom, to moral and intellectual activities through

11

which humans realize their essence and stabilize society (cf. Aristotle, 1998, X.6, 1177a, pp. 20–1).

Communication theorists and mainstream engineers have embraced the instrumentalist tradition, for example, Negroponte's (1996) *Being Digital*. For the inventor of cybernetics, Wiener (1948, 1954), politicians should fret over technology's impact, but allow engineers efficiency in the laboratory. For Shannon and Weaver (1949), it provides a framework for statistical models of media transmission that inspire our inventions from 60,000 bits per second in telephone wires to 100 billion bits per second in light-based fiber optics.

The legacy of tools as neutral is a placid, clean, and congenial model. But when working on global media ethics, this instrumentalist definition of technology is inadequate and unacceptable for three reasons:

1. The technical definition excludes engineers and scientists from responsibility. It allows them to be technical experts and wizards at engineering but with tunnel vision. They need not worry about results. Steve Jobs and Bill Gates ought not to be questioned; responsibility rests with journalists who are madly switching to online technology. Under this view, if YouTube is used to ridicule people instead of build friendships, if television is excessively violent, and if catastrophic climatic changes occur because of too much carbon dioxide in the atmosphere, the persons who created these technological products should not be blamed. Responsibility rests with politicians, a greedy sales force, journalists, and individual consumers for the use they make of them. However, instead of excusing engineers and inventors, we ought to hold their feet to the fire.

2. The instrumental philosophy of technology promotes virtuosity values. It channels our intellectual energy and financial resources into high technology, into improving the performance of tools. Virtuosity allows unchallenged the myth of the technological sublime. But we need a definition in which the "technically sweet" is eliminated in favor of user values—maintenance, prevention, husbandry of natural resources, dependability, and disposability.

3. A narrow definition of technology advocates the technical fix. Better professions are said to require better tools. Social improvement, civilization's future, and society's problems are gathered around a technological product or tool. The technical fix seeks to solve a problem by technique alone. Chemical water treatment is used for river pollution. Computers are put in schools rather than making broad changes, including more and better-trained teachers and smaller classes.

The neutral model is the instrumentalist mind at work. Instead of minor adjustments in the instrumental model, we need to reconceive technology itself. Transmission theories of neutral media defend a particular social philosophy, that is, instrumentalism. And over a theory of society the battle ought to be waged. Pleading for changes here and there is futile. The epistemology of the neutral view is wrong. The whole phenomenon ought to be called into question, not just some of its features. A fundamentally different approach to technology is necessary.

The philosophical literature on technology develops an important critique of the neutrality view. Wajcman's (1991) *Feminism Confronts Technology* and her *Techno-Feminism* (2004) demonstrate how the instrumental view of technology allows for gender discrimination. Feenberg's (1991) classic *A Critical Theory of Technology* and his *Transforming Technology* (2002) argue that technology as a neutral tool pushes social change to the margins. Regarding the questions of media ethics, an uncritical acceptance of neutrality leaves fundamental matters of morality unaddressed. Freedom and responsibility are primary. The ethical domain is meaningless if moral choices are not made without coercion. Without accountability, professional standards, principles, and codes of ethics are ephemeral. The neutrality view presumes that neither freedom nor responsibility is a problem when philosophical reflection indicates otherwise.

First, freedom. Our standard approach to freedom is political. The media need freedom from government control—from censorship—to serve the public responsibly. Both negative and positive freedom in Berlin's (1990) *Four Essays on Liberty* are political in orientation. While not denying the importance of political freedom and freedom from the market, the philosophy of technology worries about a deeper and more complicated loss of freedom through instrumentalism. This is a universe of necessity, not just a world of technological artifacts. The problem is the dominance of technical modes of thought over the human orders of culture, morality, politics, and education. When we claim ultimacy and universality for technology, and worship it as unassailable, then its necessary character is most dramatic. We imbue technology with an aura of holy prestige, and it is this aggrandizement that enslaves us.

As the media open up our horizons, determine our conversations, and shape our self-identity, they foster a technicized view of life—what Ellul (1954) calls *la technique*. If the massive state and world-wide industrial order are *la technique*'s supreme embodiments, communication systems are its innermost manifestation. The media, themselves co-opted by instrumentalism, do not transmit neutral messages but subtly weave users and society into the warp and woof of an efficiency-dominated culture. In Baudrillard's (1983) *Simulations*, the enormous development of media technologies has shifted modern civilization from production to reproduction. Humans become modules in electronic networks. We create cybernetic models to organize our experience, but a reversal occurs and reality arises from them instead. The world of electronic codes, the hyperreal, implodes and becomes reality. Whatever can be digitalized and codified is considered definitive. We follow the technological imperative instead of ethics. Technology tells us what news should be, what kinds of advertising campaigns ought to be designed, and what entertainment programs can be distributed most effectively.

If we presume that we only need to eliminate defective parts, or balance political and economic disproportions, or fill visible gaps, we will pursue these reforms, rather than seriously engage the pervasive malaise of our time. Technology removes humankind's ancient constraints, but it does not make us free. Destruction of *la technique*, rather than the reform of technological products and practices, must be the starting point of change. Finding freedom in a technological civilization is in essence a philosophical problem. Unable to distinguish a meaningful life outside the artificial ambience of a technological culture, human beings place their ultimate hope in it. Seeing no other source of security, and failing to recognize the illusoriness of their technical autonomy, they become slaves to the exactitude of mechanical systems. Ellul opposes the powerful phenomenon of machineness as a dehumanizing force and exposes it as contrary to the norms of love and justice.

Second, regarding responsibility, instrumentalism fails to see the turn to amorality in technological regimes. The instrumentalism driving the technological age subverts our ability to make moral judgments. A calculus of averages and probabilities replaces ends and the common good. The technological order reconstitutes the moral order in terms of technique. Human ends are buried under a preoccupation with means. Efficiency and morality are a contradiction in terms. The moral life is alien, moral vocabulary cannot be heard or understood.

In domains of technicism, we face a crisis—not the violation of norms, first of all, but the vacuum of normlessness. Moral distinctions have little meaning. Calls for justice cannot be heard clearly in a technocratic culture. Justice is basic to the social order, and fundamental to a global media ethics. But even modernist justice as fairness has been emaciated by the crises of contemporary life. It is haunted by its inability to determine criteria for inequality, its struggles over which kind of inequalities beyond income matter, and how far inequalities should go. In technological nations, such as the United States when debating health-care reform, the basic justice of including everyone in health care is not presumed but ignored or considered debatable. In the highly technological regime we call the mass media, ethics is typically considered an intrusion on the media's neutrality.

Human-centered Philosophy of Technology

To orient media ethics in the right direction, a different philosophy of technology is essential. Rather than be content with critique only, and live with the traditional dualism of means and ends, the instrumentalist worldview needs to be confronted head on.

Heidegger's Dasein

By examining technology philosophically, Martin Heidegger (1889–1976) destroys the instrumentalist paradigm. In contrast to the traditional conception, technology for Heidegger (1977b) is an ontological issue. Humans do not stand outside technology, but technology is intertwined with the existential structure of human being. The foundations of the technological enterprise are rooted in human life. The meaning of technology is known through the way it works itself into our humanness.

Human beingness (Dasein, "therebeing") is not a static substance, but a phenomenon of its location in history. The technological era does not exist external to human beings, but is their home. Technology and human being stir through one another like a giant food mixer. Rather than homo faber (humans as tool makers to meet basic needs such as food and shelter), our being is understood only through the technological phenomenon. Technology is not mere means or products, but a mode of revealing humanness. Humans as living beings exist within a historical and sociological framework. Beings as such are never simply given. Technology is not an individual invention, but takes shape within assumptions about the world that are taken for granted. In the contemporary age, the creation of technologies takes place under conditions of scientific and commercial prowess, rationalism, and secularism. Our life-world has a technological texture that stipulates for us what existence means. In Heidegger's terms, the modern epoch is technological, and Being is technicized as a result.

Media technologies are especially powerful mechanisms for reconstructing an inauthentic humanness. In this mediated process of enculturation, commonplaces and conformity bubble up from below to homogenize rather than inform. Viewers and readers are cast up as purchasers. Private and confidential data become commodities for digital information banks. In genetic engineering, humans are raw material, fodder for scientific experimentation. Relentlessly and overwhelmingly, the technological process pre-empts human existence for itself. The challenge of convergent media in a technological age can only be met by a new worldview.

The Tao of Physics

Heidegger's philosophy of human-centered technology has a German cadence, but it speaks about our humanity as a whole. Preceding the industrial world that Heidegger addressed, Taoism made our humanness non-negotiable. Great ideas are seldom unique; they surface in several places when conditions and needs trigger their visibility. Accordingly, Heidegger is not a European landmark for the world to emulate, but a German variant of a need in technological regimes for a humano-centric philosophy of technology. In fact, Heidegger's interest in Eastern thought, and the symmetry between his Dasein and the Tao are well known (May, 1996; Parkes, 1990). Kakuzo's concept of *das-in-der-Welt-sein* (being in the world) to describe Buddhist thinking was given to Heidegger in 1919 by a Buddhist scholar studying with him. In Chang's terms, "Heidegger is the only Western philosopher who not only intellectually but has intuitively grasped Taoist thought" (1963, p. 190).[1]

In *The Tao of Physics*, physicist Capra (2000) establishes parallels between quantum physics as a science and Eastern philosophies. He works on the big-picture level, seeing similar ideas in both: the interrelation of all things and events, process as primary, symmetry between cyclotrons and mysticism, and the absence of foundational matter.

While Capra seeks a philosophical underpinning for modern mathematical science, a perspective on media technology is opened up by Gunaratne's "humanocentric theory of journalism" in his *The Dao of the Press* (2005). He integrates Western epistemology with Eastern mysticism to replace the media's individualism and self-interest with interdependence and mutual causality. Instead of grounding our theories of communication in politics or economics or machines, Gunaratne appeals to the human instead. In order that Eurocentrism and universalism are not *de facto* understood as one and the same, living systems for him is the integrating idea (also see Capra, 1997).

Gunaratne includes an excursus on Confucian humanism (chapter 2), but Taoism's understanding of living systems has center stage (especially chapters 1 and 5). Taoism recognizes a mysterious power in nature, and pursues the harmonious state of being united with nature. In terms of Lao Tzu's *Tao Te Ching* (2010), "Tao cannot be heard, cannot be seen, cannot be told, and should not be named." For him, Tao is a formless mysticism that gives life to all creation and is itself inexhaustible. Tao is an energy that guides human action. Tao is within persons and when humans embody it the Self gradually evolves.

From Taoism's perspective, the basic question is how we can live harmoniously in the midst of social orders and values that tend to make human beings soulless objects. Chuang Tzu contends that humans suffer because they have no freedom (1964). We lack freedom because we are attached to material goods, to feelings, knowledge and religions. Taoism advocates harmony within us and with nature in the midst of the dominant voices touting efficiency, structure and progress. It turns people's eyes to the state of life, being at one with the world. The crisis we face in technological regimes such as nations, and in professions such as journalism and advertising, is not machines and products *per se*, but a technological understanding of Being. The challenge is a philosophy of technology that is radically human to prevent totalizing closure of our humanity into technique.

Dwelling is one issue common to both, that is, living in community, feeling at home, settled. To dwell, to be set at peace, means to remain at peace within the preserve, the free sphere that safeguards each thing in its preserve: "the fundamental character of dwelling is sparing" (Heidegger, 1977a, p. 327). Dwelling means the coming together of earth, being, and divinity, with nature playing an especially active role in Taoism (Huang, 1967).[2] Instrumentalism cuts us loose from our human habitat in time and space; it pushes us away from a meditative "dwelling" toward a frenetic "doing." The result in technological regimes is the plight of undwelling or what Meyrowitz (1985) calls "the homeless mind." In a technical artifice, where is harmony with nature or within us? The worldview of efficiency that drives rapid modernization buries the emotional experience of memory, safety, peace, and rootedness. Caught up in the instrumentalism of technological regimes, their professionals and executives are harassed into hurried, technical decisions. In the original Greek, ethics is ethos, abode, dwelling, place, the human domain for moral discernment. Homelessness, no fixed abode, means the absence of ethics or moral indifference. We demand from the universe rather than live in harmony with it. As Heidegger puts it, "only if we are capable of dwelling, only then can we build" (1977a, p. 338).

Application

How can a human-centered philosophy of technology be put to work? How does it apply to professional ethics, especially the project of ethical universals? How can our theoretical models value human welfare instead of promoting instrumental efficiency? Three applications are suggestive.

Humanistic Universals

A universal theory cannot be a system of conduct binding on all rational creatures, the content of which is ascertainable by human reason. The Western modernist project to establish categorical imperatives as everywhere and always the same is discredited. The Enlightenment's abstractions, its principlism, are unacceptable. Theories of media ethics that are credible transnationally ought to be ontological instead, constitutive of our humanness.

As an alternative to anthroprocentric ethics, Gunkel (2007) proposes a machinic ethics in an age of robots, cyborgs and artificial intelligence. Mainstream conceptions of morality consist of systematic rules that can be encoded to direct behavior and govern conduct. In his view, why then should we consider thinking machines to be outside moral reasoning. The argument from the philosophy of technology goes like this: in technological regimes such as the media, all theories and practices ought to go through a human-centered understanding of technology, and a machinic ethics does not meet this test.

On the other hand, one theoretical model compatible with human-centered technology is the sacredness of human life as a universal proto-norm. This is an ontological ethics, an ethics of being, that affirms reverence for life on earth as the rationale for ethical decision-making. The sacredness of life grounds a responsibility that is global in scope and self-evident regardless of cultures and competing ideologies. This is a different kind of universal, one that honors the splendid variety of human life while articulating cross-cultural norms. Its universal scope enables us to avoid the divisiveness of appeals to individual interests, cultural practices, and national prerogatives. In Martin Luther King's proverb, "The arc of the moral universe is long, and it bends toward justice."[3] Under the instrumental approach, the arcs are straight-line abstractions as a longitude and latitude grid. The Heidegger–Tao tradition validates King's "bending toward justice."

Alternative Technologies

As a result of foregrounding technology philosophically, the speed, shape, size, and character of technology are important issues for analysis and application. Rather than focusing on the global media giants and designing ethical models only for the monopolies and big-brand media, alternative technologies that are close to the ground are of special importance. Instrumentalism thrives in big systems, and assuming they alone need to be transformed indicates that our theorizing has been co-opted by *la technique*. One inescapable question ought to be: in addition to addressing global media, does our universal theory appropriately serve community media in local cultures?

The human-centered philosophy of technology makes alternative technologies important, what the Latin Americanist Illich (1973) calls Tools for Conviviality. They are responsibly limited and empowering to the local community. Convivial technology respects the dignity of human work, needs little specialized training to operate, and is generally accessible. Convivial tools with a human face are interactive and maintain a kind of open-ended conversation with their users. Because of their simplicity and transparency, they allow community voices to speak rather than experts trained in sophisticated instruments. Independent film companies, underground presses, community radio, and popular theater can provide a competitive media system from below. Manifestoes, pamphlets from non-governmental organizations, websites, online journalism, smart phones, discussion guides, digital cameras—all in the vernacular tongue can help people movements gain their own voice and nurture appropriate options for social change. Obviously macro-systems need a media ethics that speaks to them, but alternative media do so as well. A community-oriented media ethics can play a leadership role in taking diversity and pluralism seriously.

The philosophy of technology in Heidegerrian terms insists on a media ethics that is international, but since we live in communities and practice our professions within them, such a media ethics needs to work effectively on the ground. Obviously not all communities or professional practices are morally upright; therefore standards from the outside are needed to establish local guidelines.[4] Rather than stopping with universalist general-izations, universal principles become a crucial step toward a media ethics that is actionable and pluralistic. Enlightenment-style universals imposed uniformity, but the universals advocated here do not. Through universal norms we object to communal values that are exclusionary and oppressive, and in the process we open pathways that are morally acceptable. Ethical theory needs to be thick enough to enable us to think globally and act locally at the same time.

Education

There is no technological fix or magic answer for technicism. We need to desacralize technology and free our language from technological metaphors. Given Heidegger's (1971) longstanding interest in language, he sees hope only in educational terms. This move is concentrated on a revival of art and the primal role of the poet. "Poetically man dwells upon the earth" (Heidegger, 1977b, p. 34). Art's mode of revealing "opens up new ways of 'saying Being,' as Heidegger puts it" (Idhe, 1979, p. 115). As human creations, art and engineering are similar in kind, with art "akin to the essence of technology on the one hand, and on the other, fundamentally different from it" (Heidegger, 1977b, p. 35). There are two contrasting ways of revealing. Poetry opens a new world. Technology converts the universe of being into "standing reserve" (*Bestand*) for mechanistic initiatives. Genuine art enriches human existence, while technological creation pre-empts being for itself. Against an overweening technocratic mystique, an educational culture must be developed in which questions of meaning, life's purpose, and moral values predominate.

Technological regimes face a deep emptiness, an uprootedness, a spiritual longing that has its source in technological abundance. Within a technological artifice, humans are disposed to relax or abolish the limits on their finitude. It is true that technology has limits, but from the standpoint of *la technique* itself, these limits are an affront—something to be overcome. Limits are an obstacle to be eliminated by invention and productivity.

In technological regimes driven by instrumentalism, we live with a half-truth about technology. We recognize our limitless desire to understand and control, but deny the limits on which the meaning of this desire depends. A culture of machineness encourages ignorance about ourselves. Humans seek meaning to their mortality. But our striving for the infinite as humans only has meaning within the framework of mortality. Humans yearn to be more than they are, but within the human condition where our finitude is unchanging from birth to death.

We need the humanities to develop the human condition in a technological age that obscures it from view. For a humanocentric philosophy of technology to anchor our global media ethics, our support of the humanities is indispensable. Education focuses our attention on the values that drive the technological order—calling for a transformation in our commitments to them. And only when these values, these dimensions of the instrumental worldview are revolutionized, will radical changes occur in technological regimes.

Conclusion

From the philosophy-of-technology perspective, the primordial issues in global media ethics can never be solved once-and-for-all. Given the complexity of communication ethics in a media regime governed by the technological imperative, no one academic or media professional is competent to address these issues singlehandedly. Scholarship is a shared enterprise, and this collaboration must ensure that moral philosophy in all phases is humanocentric—in metaethics, and also in normative and descriptive ethics. Education focuses our attention on the values that drive the technological order—calling for a transformation in our commitments to them. And only when these values, these dimensions of the instrumental worldview, are revolutionized will radical changes occur in technological regimes.

Developing an appropriate form of universal theory for media ethics is nearly impossible in a technocratic culture. It seems more like chasing fools gold than anything else, to construct human-centered global proto-norms, from within and on behalf of, today's global media as technological regimes. But if defensible universals are elusive or inconceivable, public communications do not have much of a future, and it is fatalism not to try.

The overwhelming power of instrumentalism tends to trap electronic technologies such as broadcasting, and now new digital media, within its efficiency, making us satisfied with means rather than ends. But a human-centered philosophy of technology does emerge on occasion from quality professionals, media executives, and academics. Both ethical theories and professional practices are a democratic resource when they are inspired by philosophical reflection in a technological age.

NOTES

1. As adopted here, most scholars see Heidegger's phenomenology and Taoist thought as illuminating each other. However, for the record, a few have argued against mutuality. Contrary to Heidegger's phenomenal existence, it is claimed, phenomenal existence in Buddhism is illusory. Moreover, it is said by a few that Lao Tzu speaks in opposition to Heidegger's "language the house of being;" being only exists because of its opposite, non-being.

2. Taoist "dwelling" is described in a fifth-century Chinese landscape poem by Hsieh Ling-yun (Huang, 1967; see also Haar and Lilly, 1993).

3. First used in 1961 and on several occasions until his last sermon, given at the National Cathedral, on May 31, 1968, four days before his death.

4. Having community life judged by universal norms follows the intellectual strategy of Habermas (1984). For an ethics of discourse to operate effectively in the public sphere, he presumed an ideal speech situation as its context. Presuming an inherent desire in speech acts for mutual understanding, Habermas argues for an ideal speech formulation of full participation, mutuality and reciprocity as a goal for citizens and a critical standard by which to judge consensus. Universals are the bridging principle which makes agreement possible (Habermas, 1990, pp. 57–68).

REFERENCES

ARISTOTLE (1998) *The Nicomachean Ethics*, W. D. Ross (Trans.), New York: Oxford University Press.

BAUDRILLARD, JEAN (1983) *Simulations*, Paul Foss, Paul Patton and Philip Beitchman (Trans.), New York: Semiotext(e).

BERLIN, ISAIAH (1990) *Four Essays on Liberty*, New York: Oxford University Press.

CAPRA, FRITJOF (1997) *The Web of Life: a scientific understanding of living systems*, New York: Random House/Anchor.

CAPRA, FRITJOF (2000) *The Tao of Physics: an exploration of the parallels between modern physics and Eastern mysticism*, 4th edn, Boston: Shambhala.

CHANG, CHUNG-YUAN (1963) *Creativity and Taoism*, New York: Julien Press.

COMMERS, M. S. RONALD, VANDEKERCKHOVE, WIM and VERLINDEN, AN (Eds) (2008) *Ethics in an Era of Globalization*, Aldershot: Ashgate.

ELLUL, JACQUES (1954) *The Technological Society*, J. Wilkinson (Trans.), New York: Random Vintage.

FEENBERG, ANDREW (1991) *A Critical Theory of Technology*, New York: Oxford University Press.

FEENBERG, ANDREW (2002) *Transforming Technology: a critical theory revisited*, 2nd edn, New York: Oxford University Press.

GUNARATNE, SHELTON (2005) *The Dao of the Press: a humanocentric theory*, Cresskill, NJ: Hampton Press.

GUNKEL, DAVID (2007) *Thinking Otherwise: philosophy, communication, technology*, Lafayette, IN: Purdue University Press.

HAAR, MICHAEL and LILLY, REGINALD (1993) *The Song of the Earth: Heidegger and the grounds of the history of being*, R. Lilly (Trans.), Bloomington: University of Indiana Press.

HABERMAS, JURGEN (1984) *The Theory of Communicative Action, Vol. 1, Reason and the rationalization of society*, T. McCarthy (Trans.), Boston: Beacon Press.

HABERMAS, JURGEN (1990) *Moral Consciousness and Communicative Action*, C. Lenhardt and S. W. Nicholsen (Trans.), Cambridge, MA: MIT Press.

HEIDEGGER, MARTIN (1971) *Poetry, Language, Thought*, A. Hofstadter (Trans.), New York: Harper & Row.

HEIDEGGER, MARTIN (1977a) "Building Dwelling Being", in: *Basic Writings*, D. F. Krell (Trans.), New York: Harper and Row, pp. 319–39.

HEIDEGGER, MARTIN (1977b) *The Question Concerning Technology and Other Essays*, W. Lovitt (Trans.), New York: Harper and Row.

HUANG, CHIEH (1967) *Hsieh K'ang-lo Shih-chu commentary on the poems of Hsieh K'ang-lo*, Taipei: Yi-wen.

IHDE, DON (1979) *Technics and Praxis*, Dordrecht: D. Reidel.

ILLICH, IVAN (1973) *Tools for Conviviality*, New York: Harper and Row.

MAY, REINHARD (1996) *Heidegger's Hidden Sources: East-Asian influences on his work*, G. Parkes (Trans.), London: Routledge.

MEYROWITZ, JOSHUA (1985) *No Sense of Place: the impact of media on social behavior*, New York: Oxford University Press.

NEGROPONTE, NICHOLAS (1996) *Being Digital*, New York: Random House Vintage.

PACEY, ARNOLD (1996) *The Culture of Technology*, Cambridge, MA: MIT Press.

PARKES, GRAHAM (Ed.) (1990) *Heidegger and Asian Thought*, Honolulu: University of Hawaii Press.

SHANNON, CLAUDE and WEAVER, WARREN (1949) *Mathematical Theory of Communication*, Urbana: University of Illinois Press.

TZU, CHUANG (1964) *Chuang Zu: basic writings*, B. Watson (Trans.), New York: Columbia University Press.

TZU, LAO (2010) *Tao Te Ching: the book of the way*, D. Goddard (Trans.), New York: Amazon Create Space.

WAJCMAN, JUDY (1991) *Feminism Confronts Technology*, New York: Polity Press.

WAJCMAN, JUDY (2004) *TechnoFeminism*, New York: Polity Press.

WIENER, NORBERT (1948) *Cybernetics or Control and Communication in the Animal and the Machine*, New York: Wiley & Sons.

WIENER, NORBERT (1954) *The Human Use of Human Beings: cybernetics and society*, 2nd edn, New York: Doubleday/Anchor.

ETHICAL FLOURISHING AS AIM OF GLOBAL MEDIA ETHICS

Stephen J. A. Ward

This paper proposes a new and comprehensive goal for global media ethics—the promotion of ethical flourishing across borders. The ideal of ethical flourishing underwrites more specific global principles and provides a target at which responsible global journalism can aim. A major task of global media ethics is to re-conceive journalism ethics around the idea of ethical flourishing. Promoting ethical flourishing is defined as the development of four levels of essential goods that together constitute the idea of the human good: individual goods, social goods, political goods, and ethical goods (or the goods of justice). These goods contribute to a life that has rational, social, political, and ethical dignity. The paper uses work in development theory and Sen's "capacity" theory to identify basic capacities that cross borders and should be protected and promoted by global media.

The reasonable generates itself and answers itself in kind. (John Rawls, 2001, p. 196)

Introduction

"Human excellence grows like a vine tree, fed by the green dew, raised up, among wise men and just, to the liquid sky."[1] So wrote the Greek poet Pindar. He knew what excellence requires. Not just innate talent but a supportive environment, including wise and just citizens. For the lack of such environment, Plato turned away from politics to philosophy, imagining an ideal Republic. Since Plato, describing a society that is both flourishing and just has been a goal of both ethical thought and social reform.

In this paper, I sketch my vision of human flourishing, described in the broadest of philosophical terms and based on my work in global journalism ethics (Ward and Wasserman, 2010). I argue that we should re-conceive journalism ethics around the idea of ethical flourishing, as one interpretation of the human good. I start by explaining the concept of ethical flourishing and develop its meaning in terms of four levels of goods. Then I will consider some implications of ethical flourishing for journalism and a global media ethics.

Ethical Flourishing

The Formal Concept

Ethical flourishing is a form of flourishing. But what is flourishing? In this context, flourishing means the exercise of one's intellectual, emotional, and other capacities to a high degree in a supportive social context. Ideally, flourishing is the fullest expression of human development under favourable conditions.[2] In reality, humans flourish in varying degrees. Few people are fully flourishing. Life often goes badly; many live in desperate conditions where flourishing is a remote ideal.

The many theories of flourishing typically rely on a biological metaphor of growth and proper functioning. There is Aristotle's notion of eudaimonia as excellence—that is, the exercise of the virtues of the well-ordered, rational soul (Aristotle, 1976). There is the liberal idea of the development of free and creative individuals who, as Mill said, experiment in ways of living (Mill, 2006). Ethical flourishing builds upon this rich tradition. It goes beyond the fact that humans can develop their capacities. Any capacity or talent, from the ability to pursue goals to the emotional capacity to be loyal, can be employed for evil purposes. We do not want cruelty, blind hatred, and war-mongering to be part of our idea of flourishing. Therefore, in ethics, we stress the development of capacities that fit our sense of the ethically good life. We combine empirical knowledge about our capacities with normative views on how to use those capacities virtuously. When we exercise our capacities ethically, we can be said to flourish ethically. We enjoy such goods as trust, friendship, and right relations with others. Civility defines our social interactions.

Ethical flourishing contains three ideas: first, the moral worth of developing capacities that are essential to a decent, dignified life; second, the importance of channelling capacities toward ethical ends such as the ability to interact respectfully with others; third, the belief that, in the end, a flourishing life needs an ethical component. It cannot be a selfish or unethical life. What link exists between the ethical life and the flourishing (or happy) individual is the question put before Socrates at the start of The Republic: Is a happy life an ethical life? Or, is a just life a happy life? Despite their irrational or destructive desires, many people still seek to be who they should be. Such humans "flower" or flourish ethically, as well as physically and socially.

A theory of ethical flourishing has two parts: a theory of important goods whose realization defines what it is to flourish; and a theory of the right which deals with how conflicts between the pursuit of these goods are to be arbitrated. Ethical flourishing gives priority to the right in the sense that the pursuit of our goods occurs within the bounds of justice. Ethical flourishing is a composite good where the good and the right are as congruent as possible. To develop a theory of the right one must decide what theory of justice to adopt. It makes a great deal of difference if one embraces a libertarian or an egalitarian idea of justice.[3] So far, I have described only the formal concept of ethical flourishing. My description lacks particulars. To use Kantian language, it is a conceptual schema, an idea of reason, waiting to be filled in by more specific intuitions.

Four Levels of the Good

I give content to this schema by explaining ethical flourishing as the development of four levels of goods. The schema reflects my attempt to draw the picture of a life worthy of humans, what life can be when it goes well. I draw inspiration from ideas on human development and welfare, and by reflecting on what it is for humans to flourish. In this project I claim no originality apart from my particular systematization. I draw eclectically on ideas from many places, from Sen's "capabilities" approach (Sen, 1993, p. 30) to Nussbaum's notion of a dignified life (Nussbaum, 2006).

When I review the goods of life, I find that they can be placed into four groups—individual, social, political, and ethical. To achieve the goods of each level is to achieve a form of human dignity: individual, social, political and ethical dignity. By individual goods, I mean the goods that come from the development of each individual's capacities. By social goods, I mean those goods that come from individuals participating in society. By political goods, I mean the goods that accrue to us as citizens living in a just political association. By ethical goods, I mean the goods that come from living among persons and institutions of ethical character.

Level One, the level of individual goods, contains the physical goods that give a person physical dignity. All persons need food, shelter, and security to live a normal length of life in good health. It contains rational and moral goods allow physical capacity to flower into distinct human traits. A person enjoys the rational and moral goods when she develops her capacities to observe and think as a critical individual, and to carry out a rational plan of life. Such a person is able to form emotional attachments, and to use their imagination to produce (or enjoy) creative and intellectual works. Also, the person is able to be a moral agent. She is able to empathize with others and to form a sense of justice. She is able to deliberate about the good of others.

Level Two, the social goods, arise when we use our rational and moral capacities to participate in society. Human reality is "social" not just because, instrumentally, humans need society to develop language and culture. Humans are inherently social creatures. Humans come to value participating in common projects as a good-in-itself. Among the social goods are the freedom to enter into and benefit from economic association, the goods of love and friendship; the need for mutual recognition and respect. In this manner, we achieve a social dignity.

In addition to the social goods, there are also the political goods of Level Three. These are the goods that humans enjoy when they live in a society that has a reasonably just political structure. These goods include the basic liberties, such as freedom of speech and freedom to pursue one's goods, combined with the opportunity and resources to exercise these freedoms. Citizens are able to participate in political life, to hold office, and to influence decisions. The primary means to these public goods are constitutional protections, the rule of law, and barriers against undue coercion, and means for the peaceful resolution of disputes. A citizen who enjoys these goods has a political dignity, through self-government.

There is also a fourth level of goods, ethical goods. To enjoy a full measure of the human good we need to live not only in a society of rational people—that is, people motivated to pursue their own interests. A society motivated only by purely rational agents would be a terrifying 'private' (or extremely individualistic) society. To flourish, we also need to live among people of ethical character. These people are rational agents who are also disposed to be what Rawls (1993, p. 48) calls morally "reasonable." Reasonable citizens are motivated to consider the interests of others and the greater public good. Ethical flourishing means more than restraining our actions within laws. It indicates something positive: constructing societies where citizens come to appreciate the positive goods of justice and living in right relations. Of course, many people are not motivated to adopt the ethical stance. Nevertheless, under certain conditions, humans can appreciate interacting ethically as a good-in-itself.

My scheme is not a practical manual. It does not presume to tell development workers what day-to-day strategies to employ in underdeveloped countries. We need to distinguish between "What constitutes the ideal of ethical flourishing?" and "What should we do to help people in country x emerge from chaos and dire need?" To deal with extreme poverty in developing countries, agencies rightly focus on a small number of basic needs. However, my theory is not without some practical implications. The four levels provide criteria by which to judge development. Also, the theory suggests a two-stage approach to development in poor countries. The first stage aims at a decent and minimally flourishing life, where physical goods are primary. The second stage aims at an ethically flourishing life, not just a decent life, by developing all four levels.

This is my four-level scheme, in brief. My approach is holistic. Wherever possible, the goods of each level should be integrated and developed simultaneously. I do not pick out one good (or one level) as sufficient to define the human good, such as pleasure, or utility. The human good is a composite of basic goods, none of which are reducible or eliminable. For example, my view is not ascetic. It does not propose that the human good requires people to seek happiness by drastically reducing their desires and goods to a minimum, and to withdraw from public life and its goods. Nor does it, like libertarianism, stress the goodness of one of the political capacities—not be interfered with in exercising one's negative freedom. In my view, the satisfaction of one type of good allows another to exist. To be sure, we need to secure the physical goods before we can move on to other goods, but that does not make the other levels less important. In many countries, unstable political structures—that is, the lack of political goods—interfere with attempts to provide physical and social goods to citizens.

What is the link between ethical flourishing and global ethics? Ethical flourishing is global because it identifies goods that apply to people insofar as they are human. Ethical flourishing becomes the basis of a global ethic when we take the aim of ethical flourishing to be global ethical flourishing. It is no longer only the promotion of flourishing in Canada or China. The goal is the promotion of the four levels across borders. We improve the conditions that allow humans everywhere to pursue the four goods. The individual, social, political, and ethical dignity that we seek for citizens in our society, we seek for humanity at large. Practically, the goal is to increase the number of citizens of the world who enjoy a reasonable amount of the four levels of the good within the bounds of global justice. Ethical flourishing expresses the impulse of the ethics of cosmopolitanism, which asserts the equal value and dignity of all, as members of a common humanity (Ward and Wasserman, 2010). To work towards the ethical flourishing of a global community is to promote a cosmopolitanism that emphasizes universal principles of human rights, freedom, and justice.

Application to Journalism

Changing the Aim

I turn to the implications of ethical flourishing for journalism ethics. If we adopt ethical flourishing, we begin a chain of re-definitions and new interpretations that reverberates across the entire field of journalism ethics.

Let us start with the aims of journalism. If we adopt ethical flourishing, then the ethical aim of journalism becomes the aim of ethics understood as promoting the four levels of goods. Historically, journalism ethics has been parochial; its codes applied to particular groups. Journalism ethics was developed for a journalism of limited reach.

In the West, the aim of journalism has been described more narrowly than ethical flourishing. Typically, codes of ethics describe the aim in political terms—serving the public as self-governing citizens through accurate impartial informing, acting as a watchdog on government, and creating a forum for views. This concept of journalism's aim as serving the public good is contained in my third level of the good—the political goods.

A few years ago, I expressed this change in journalism's aims as following a number of imperatives (Ward, 2005). Journalists, I said, should see themselves as agents of a global public sphere. The goal of their collective actions is a well-informed, diverse, and tolerant global "info-sphere" that challenges the abuse of human rights. The global journalist uses a diversity of sources and perspectives to promote a nuanced understanding of issues from an international perspective. These imperatives defined what I called "the claim of humanity" on journalists.

My theory of ethical flourishing spells out in greater detail the claim of humanity. Journalism serves humanity by promoting the four levels across borders. Global journalists seek the individual, social, political, and ethical dignity for humanity at large. Journalism can promote the individual goods of Level One by monitoring basic levels of physical, individual, and social dignity. Journalists need to inquire into the effectiveness of educational and other systems in developing rational and imaginative citizens. What are the opportunities for philosophical, scientific, and cultural engagement? Also, journalists should do stories on people who have been denied physical, rational, and moral dignity, and investigate whether gender, ethnicity, and other differences account for inequalities.

Journalism can promote the social goods by reporting critically on how society structures economic associations and monitors the growth of private monopolies of power. Journalism has a duty not just to report the latest business news but to report on how society allows citizens to participate and benefit from various forms of economic association. Journalists should always ask: Who benefits from the economic status quo? Journalists also assist the social goods by providing a cultural and informational bridge between diverse classes, ethnic groups, and cultures within and among countries. Journalists should also play a key role in developing media literacy among citizens. It should inquire into the impact of journalism, media, and communication technology on society, domestic and global.

Journalism can promote the political goods by reporting on the basic political and institutional structures of society. How well are political constitutions and principles of justice embodied by institutions, political processes, and the legal system? To what extent are citizens able to enjoy the full value of basic liberties, such as freedom of speech, freedom of association, and freedom from discrimination? Journalism needs to encourage citizen participation in public life and enhance their ability to have a meaningful influence on decisions. To be sure, journalism favours a free marketplace of ideas but it should also question whether that marketplace has distortions, like all marketplaces. Is it a diverse public forum with adequate representation of non-dominant groups? What inequalities distort the public sphere when it goes global?

Also, in a pluralistic world, we need to question how public means of communication allow citizens to discuss issues. Is the public discourse too timid, or is it too much on the surface? Or is the discourse redolent with unhelpful ranting and ideology? At the core of the media system should be "deliberative spaces"—spaces where reasonable citizens can robustly but respectfully exchanges views and evaluate proposals. In a media-saturated world, the nature of media communication will largely determine progress toward or away from ethical flourishing.

Therefore at the forefront of journalism ethics is a dual task—a simultaneous commitment to liberty and equality. Journalism should support not only creative, energetic individuals, but also individuals who are reasonable citizens seeking just social arrangements. This dual task defines the contemporary meaning of the phrase, "a free and responsible press."

Adopting Cosmopolitanism

Let us now consider the sort of attitude that ethical flourishing would bring to journalism. It would bring a cosmopolitan attitude. Cosmopolitanism has features useful to global journalism ethics. As a war correspondent I was stirred by glimpses of our common humanity, as well as dismayed by what happened when we place too much emphasis on the local, on "blood and belonging." Cosmopolitanism recommends to global journalists sensitivity to humanity.

Cosmopolitanism implies that journalists accept that transnational principles of human rights and social justice take precedence over their own interests, or even the interests of their country, when they conflict (Appiah, 2006). This emphasis on what is ethically prior provides some direction to journalists caught in the ethical maze of international events. When my country embarks on an unjust war against another country, I, as a journalist (or citizen), should say so. If I am a Canadian journalist and I learn that Canada is engaged in trading practices that condemn citizens of an African country to continuing, abject poverty, I should not hesitate to report the injustice. It is not a violation of any reasonable form of patriotism or citizenship to hold one's country to higher standards. The cosmopolitan attitude limits our parochial attachments in journalism by drawing a ring of broader ethical principles around them. When there is no conflict with cosmopolitan principles, journalists can report in ways that support local and national communities. They can practice their craft parochially.

In addition, a journalism of global flourishing would work towards a de-Westernization of journalism ethics as put forward by critical, post-colonial and other reflections on media. The effect would be a widening of the whole enterprise of journalism ethics. Such theories ask: how can discussion around a global ethics be open to many perspectives, including non-Western voices and values? For example, some writers have examined whether the African tradition of ubuntuism should be the fundamental ethical value for African journalism, since ubuntuism's communal values are more in line with African society than with the Western ideal of a free press. Rao and Wasserman (2007) and others (Ward and Wasserman, 2010) speak of an ethics that benefits from a rich dialogue between the global and the local. De-Westernization means using cross-cultural comparisons when discussing and teaching the principles of media ethics, and giving due weight to African, Indian, and Eastern ethical systems.

Another implication is that journalism ethics should place more emphasis on the representation of others since misrepresentation can spark wars, demean other cultures, and support unjust social structures. Such issues go beyond factual accuracy and fairness. They require journalists to have a deeper cultural knowledge and a deeper appreciation of how language can distort the other.

Once we move theoretically in this direction, other changes follow. To start with, consider the idea of journalism's social contract. If cosmopolitan journalism has a social contract, it is not with a particular public or society; instead, it seems to be something much more diffuse—a multi-society contract. The cosmopolitan journalist is a transnational public communicator who seeks the trust and credence of a global audience. Also, the ideal of objectivity in news coverage takes on an international sense. Traditionally, news objectivity asks journalists to avoid bias toward groups within one's own country. Global objectivity would discourage allowing bias toward one's country to distort reports on international issues. The ideas of accuracy and balance also become enlarged to include reports with international sources and cross-cultural perspectives. Global journalism also asks journalists to be more conscious of how they frame major stories, how they set the international news agenda, and how they can spark violence in tense societies.

Finally, a cosmopolitan journalism must re-think the role of patriotism. I have argued for a moderate patriotism that places ethical restraints on claims of patriotism (Ward and Wasserman, 2010). At the very least, a moderate patriotism rejects dangerous, inward-looking attitudes such as xenophobia and extreme patriotism. Journalism must not participate in demonizing other groups, especially in times of tension. The duty of journalism in times of uncertainty is not a patriotism of blind allegiance or muted criticism. In such times, journalists serve their countries—that is, are patriotic—by continuing to provide independent news and analysis. This dogged determination of journalists to continue to bring a critical attitude toward their country's actions, despite the strong patriotic feelings of their fellow citizens, is an example of what the Spanish philosopher Ortega Y Gasset (2000, p. 105) has called "criticism as patriotism." Moreover, in a global world, patriotism should play an even less powerful role in our value scheme. It is possible to question the adequacy of this traditional, nation-based notion of patriotism for an evolving cosmopolitan journalism. Nation-based forms of patriotism remain ethically permissible if they do not conflict with the demands of a global ethical flourishing.

The cosmopolitan attitude does not imply that news organizations should ignore local issues or regional audiences. It does not mean that every story requires a cosmo-politan attitude. However, there are situations, such as military intervention in a foreign country, climate change, and the establishment of a fair world trading system, where we need to assess actions from a perspective of global justice and reasonableness. What is at issue is a gradual widening of basic editorial attitudes and standards—a widening of journalists' vision of their responsibilities. It asks them to consider their society's actions, policies, and values from a larger perspective.

Therefore, if you ask, "What is global journalism ethics?" my short answer is: a cosmopolitan journalism that aims at global ethical flourishing. It amounts to: (1) a reinterpretation of journalism's aims in terms of broader goals; (2) the construction of new principles as evaluative guides for global journalism plus the re-interpretation of existing ideas; and (3) the application of these ideas to the coverage of issues and events.

Conclusion

In conclusion, I address some possible misunderstandings about my project. First, what is the status of my idea of ethical flourishing? It is a proposal, asking you to consider thinking about things in a certain manner. Why do I use the language of proposal?

Because a global media ethics is not yet constructed. We are at a stage where different conceptions are possible. Therefore scholars need to put forward ideas in an experimental and non-dogmatic spirit. We need an open and rich discussion. In such a climate, the age-old philosophical posture of speaking from certain knowledge or special insight is inappropriate and unhelpful. My expectation is that, if and when a global media ethics takes definitive shape, it will be a hybrid of good ideas contributed by co-operating ethicists and journalists.

Second, my theory operates deliberately at this high level of generality so as to be a theory with a chance of crossing borders. The theory is designed to be tolerant of differences in ethics, in culture, and in media systems. The four levels can be realized in many ways and in different degrees. I also hope that the cosmopolitan attitude I advocate can be adopted by many forms of journalists, codes of ethics, and media systems.

However, my scheme is not "neutral" in the sense of not deriving its ideas from any particular tradition or set of values. It begins with the philosophical values embedded in but not limited to Western ethics. Some of the goods I mention are universal, in the sense that they are desired by every human being, such as the physical goods of security and food. Other values, like my democratic political goods, are based on the view that this is the best way to organize human life and hold out the most promise for human flourishing. Even where disagreements arise, I hope these ideas can at least prompt discussion among people from different traditions.

Finally, I am acutely aware of the limitations of ethical theory to change something as multi-faceted and economically structured as journalism, much less move the world toward a more just and sustainable planet. Yet the power of ideas works over long periods of time. It requires a degree of patience and hope. In the end, we all do what we can do. As a philosopher I plant ideas like seeds in the hope of germination down the line. Moreover, fundamental theory is especially important today when ethics is in transition, and we wish to construct a global media ethics. Rethinking basic goals is part our ability to reason and to act consistently. Without such aims, practice lacks a target at which to aim and theory lacks a standard of evaluation.

I see the construction of global media ethics as occurring on a series of levels simultaneously: the level of high theory about ultimate goals and basic principles; the level of applied ethics where "thin" abstract ethical notions of the good and the right intersect with "thicker" context-bound professional values such as news objectivity; and a third and more concrete level where these ideas are applied to practice, changing how we report on events such as an international meeting on climate change or a looming conflict between nations.

And finally, there comes a time when the theoretical desire to understand media should be expressed in terms of action and reform. Media intellectuals, media teachers, concerned citizens—all need to consider seriously current developments in global media and what might be done so that media education and media systems embrace cosmopolitan values.

NOTES

1.   Pindar, Nemean Odes, VIII, 37–44, as quoted in Nussbaum (1986, p. vi).
2.   Aristotle was one of the first philosophers to apply this biological perspective to the analysis of the good life. In modern ethical theory, the concept of flourishing received

special attention in Anscombe (1997). The concept appears in many other works such as Nussbaum (2006), Brink (1989), Sen (1993), and Kraut (2007).

3.   See, for example, the differences between the egalitarian theory of justice of John Rawls (2001) and the libertarian idea of justice in Nozick (1974).

REFERENCES

ANSCOMBE, GERTRUDE E. M. (1997) "Modern Moral Philosophy", in: Roger Crisp and Michael Slote (Eds), *Virtue Ethics*, Oxford: Oxford University Press, pp. 26–44.

APPIAH, KWAME ANTHONY (2006) *Cosmopolitanism: ethics in a world of strangers*, New York: Norton.

ARISTOTLE (1976) *The Ethics of Aristotle: the Nicomachean ethics*, J. A. K. Thomson (Trans.), London: Penguin.

BRINK, DAVID O. (1989) *Moral Realism and the Foundations of Ethics*, Cambridge: Cambridge University Press.

KRAUT, RICHARD (2007) *What Is Good and Why: the ethics of well-being*, Cambridge, MA: Harvard University Press.

MILL, JOHN STUART (2006) *On Liberty and the Subjection of Women*, Alan Ryan (Ed.), London: Penguin Books.

NOZICK, ROBERT (1974) *Anarchy, State, and Utopia*, New York: Basic Books.

NUSSBAUM, MARTHA C. (1986) *The Fragility of Goodness: luck and ethics in Greek tragedy and philosophy*, rev. edn, Cambridge: Cambridge University Press.

NUSSBAUM, MARTHA C. (2006) *Frontiers of Justice*, Cambridge, MA: Belknap Press.

ORTEGA Y GASSET, JOSE (2000) *Meditations on Quixote*, Evelyn Rugg and Diego Marin (Trans.), Urbana and Chicago: University of Illinois Press.

RAO, SHAKUNTALA and WASSERMAN, HERMAN (2007) "Global Media Ethics Revisited: a postcolonial critique", *Global Media and Communication* 3(1), pp. 29–50.

RAWLS, JOHN (1993) *Political Liberalism*, New York: Columbia University Press.

RAWLS, JOHN (2001) *Justice as Fairness: a restatement*, Erin Kelly (Ed.), Cambridge, MA: Harvard University Press.

SEN, AMARTYA (1993) "Capability and Well-being", in: Martha Nussbaum and Amartya Sen (Eds), *The Quality of Life*, Oxford: Clarendon Press, pp. 30–61.

WARD, STEPHEN J. A. (2005) "Philosophical Foundations for Global Journalism Ethics", *Journal of Mass Media Ethics* 20(1), pp. 3–21.

WARD, STEPHEN J. A. and WASSERMAN, HERMAN (2010) "Towards an Open Ethics: implications of new media platforms for global ethics discourse", *Journal of Mass Media Ethics* 24(4), pp. 275–92.

CONTESTING PATRIOTISM AND GLOBAL JOURNALISM ETHICS IN ARAB JOURNALISM

Abeer Al-Najjar

Journalists' understanding of patriotism seems to be contextual, varies across time and depends on specific cultural and political situations. This paper investigates how global ethical journalism standards of impartiality and objectivity are challenged by patriotism among Arab journalists. It discusses two case studies: the coverage of Al-Jazeera news channel of the War on Gaza and the Egyptian media coverage of the aftermath of the World Cup qualifying football match between the Egyptian and Algerian national teams. Both cases show that patriotism, for many Arab journalists, is a virtue and not a breach of journalism ethics though journalists also believe that such patriotism could stifle criticism of the current political order and lack of press freedom.

Introduction

This essay examines the reasons that hamper Arab journalists' adoption and endorsement of Western-oriented global journalistic ethics, especially in relation to patriotism. There are many challenges that Arab journalists face as they produce their news stories and develop their professional values. This paper argues that numerous factors are worth considering in the examination of patriotism in Arab journalism. The first is the lack of efficacy of Western journalistic ethics when it comes to reporting the Palestinian–Israeli conflict as asymmetrical. Second, journalists have to appease both public and government in their professional conduct. Third, patriotism seems to be viewed as a virtue among many Arab audiences, journalists, and government officials. Hence, the meanings, value, and practicality of non-biased reporting could be contested. Impartiality does not seem to be understood as an undisputed ethical ideal for Arab journalists, especially when their own countries are involved in the conflict. Two cases are examined in this paper: Qatar-based Al-Jazeera network's coverage of the Palestinian–Israeli conflict, particularly the War on Gaza between December 2008 and January 2009; and the Egyptian media coverage of the World Cup qualifying match between the Egyptian and Algerian national teams on November 18, 2009.

Patriotism and Journalism

The Stanford Encyclopedia of Philosophy defines patriotism as "love of one's country, identification with it, and special concern for its well-being and that of compatriots" (Primoratz, 2009). Love and loyalty seem to be integral components of patriotism (Tan, 2004). Patriotism is the awareness of our moral duties to a political community

(Acton, 1972, p. 163). The morality and value of patriotism is argued and contested amongst scholars and philosophers. This contestation largely depends on the various interpretations of its very nature. MacIntyre (1984) thinks that patriotism is in contrast of a person's commitment to ethics and moral principles. Kateb postulates that, as a matter of principle, patriotism is a "mistake ... It is typically a grave moral error and its source is typically a state of mental confusion" (2006, p. 3). It is hard to differentiate between "moderate" patriotism and a more "harmful national chauvinism" (Primoratz, 2009).

The meaning, interpretation, and moral judgment of patriotism at a certain historical moment could be contextual and highly contested. Patriotism seems to be more controversial for journalists since their professional ethics requires a level of detachment, balance, impartiality, fairness, and independence (Ericson, 1988). The principle of impartiality seems to be at odds with patriotism, since the latter necessitates to side with the journalist's own country, people, or national interests. The relationship between patriotism and "truth-telling journalism" is "difficult" (Murphy et al., 2006, p. 323). Although, the writers consider the value of patriotism's qualities, they still recognize the fact that it does not safeguard news against imminent ideological bias. Thus, "genuine conscientiousness in the pursuit of truth demands higher order virtues, such as impartiality, humility, courage, and a willingness to follow the facts where they lead" (Murphy et al., 2006, p. 326).

For journalists, journalism is the independent voice and one that represents the audiences (Elliott, 2004). In ethical deliberations, journalists take into account many "considerations" and beliefs, for example "the principle of the good, the right and the virtuous" (Ward, 2007, p. 182). Ward recognizes patriotism as one of the most important challenges to global ethical journalistic practices and he suggests a "moderate" or "democratic patriotism" (2010, p. 213) that is "open to the force of reason and facts" (2010, p. 214). Moderate patriotism excludes all types of blind loyalty to the leader and its main focus is democratic institutions, system, or participation. Even in Western democracies where professional journalism ethics is highly valued and where freedom of speech is often guaranteed in Constitutions, patriotism can sometimes be viewed as a virtue, especially in times of conflict. The type of patriotism that journalists tend to display in those circumstances make them "narrow and non-democratic" (Ward, 2010, p. 213). For instance, post-9/11 for a US journalist to be seen as unpatriotic would have made the person an outcast (Salaita, 2005).

The State of Arab Journalism: Freedom of the Press, Independence and Other Challenges to Professionalism and Ethical Practices

Prior to the satellite television revolution, Arab journalists had depended on Western sources, news agencies and press for news, even about their own countries (Mellor, 2009). It was not until the late 1990s, and particularly after Al-Jazeera was formed in 1996, that Arab news media started to become an important and relevant source of news for Arab audiences. Al-Jazeera has made "tremendous inroads into the Western-dominated flow of news" (Hafez, 2005). Arab journalists also faced significant challenges in their professional performance. These challenges were: lack of freedom of the press in their respective countries, lack of security when doing their jobs, and the environment in which they worked. Mellor writes, "The political environment of the Arab world and the prevalence of authoritarian regimes in most of the Arab states have certainly resulted in censorship and control of the Arab press and broadcasting" (2009, p. 318). Though resisted by many journalists, Arab governments continue to control and censor the media, labeling it as a "form of civic responsibility" (Amin, 2001, p. 24). By this officials mean being responsible towards governmental officials and accountable against the ideals they set for good journalism.

Although Arab journalists are not a homogenous body of professionals, we still can speak of common cultural elements and political conditions. For instance, journalists could be subjected to punishment from the state or become victims of violence perpetrated by non-governmental extremist groups (Fandy, 2007). Being critical of the government or one of these political or religious actors can cost the journalist his or her life. Examples include the disappearance of journalist Rida Hilal from Egypt; the assassination of *Le Monde* journalist Samir Qaseer; and assassination of Gibran Tueni, the editor of *Al-Nahar* newspaper in Lebanon. Many journalists have been killed in wars in Iraq, Palestine, Lebanon, Sudan, and Yemen. Besides the dangers they face of getting targeted or arbitrarily killed in Iraq, they were often subjected to public anger (Badrakhan, 2006). Many journalists have been held without charges, as in the case of Yemeni journalists. In Syria, for instance, journalist Nizar Nayuf was sentenced to 10 years imprisonment on ridiculous charges of "advocating human rights" according to the Syrian Human Rights Committee (2001).

The Syndicate of Arab Journalists, in their annual meeting in Tunis in 2010, reported that Arab journalists suffer from various degrees of restrictions and threats that jeopardize their journalistic freedom. The Syndicate criticized the legal framework within which journalists perform their jobs, indicating that "it fails to provide journalists with the minimal personal or professional security guarantees" (Al-Bawaba, 2010, p. 11). In Reporters Without Borders' *Press Freedom Index* of 2010, Lebanon had the highest rank amongst Arab countries as number 78 in 178 countries, falling 17 spots from last year's report. Moreover, other Arab countries such as Sudan, Yemen, and Syria were ranked as having the least press freedom in the world (Reporters Without Borders, 2010). Many of the Arab journalists are very aware of problems in the way Arab media functions. Almost half of the sample of Arab journalists surveyed by Pintak and Ginges reported that the "independence" of their own media organizations from government manipulation was "poor" and 40 percent of the journalists viewed professionalism of Arab media "poor" as well (2009, pp. 161–2). Rami Khouri, executive editor of the Beirut-based *Daily Star* newspaper asserts that Arab media produces "extreme expressions of political sentiments and polarization" (Al-Arian, 2004).

Arab Journalists, Patriotism and Global Journalism Ethics

In many of the professional associations of Arab journalists, patriotism is understood as a quality. The draft code of the 1996 Egyptian Press Syndicate requires the news media to "adhere to the patriotic and moral values of the Egyptian society" (Hafez, 2002, p. 236). Similarly, the Lebanese *Charter of Professional Honor and the Code of Information* (Nordenstreng, 1989, pp. 177–8) makes positive references to nationalism and patriotism. In Algeria, journalists are asked to remain loyal to "the objectives of the Algerian Revolution" (Mellor, 2005, p. 33). Impartial journalism is usually discussed as being possible and feasible only in a democratic society. Impartiality is portrayed to serve certain set of interests, values, and meanings that are culturally grounded and are tailored to facilitate democracy. The audiences are citizens; journalists report news on a democratically elected government or president and other institutions within this political model and culture. In this context, freedom of the press is a well-established value to which the government, media, public, and all social and political institutes and actors are committed. In the Arab region, the political models are different. Impartial and objective journalism can be very costly for the journalist since it can lead to punishment and criticism. Essentially, ethical journalism is seen as one that tends to support the existing political and social setting making patriotism a desirable virtue. In developing any sense of global journalism ethics, Ward (2004) has suggested professional and ethical evolution of a "global journalism". For him local journalists must develop an appreciation of the "global journalist" and that local ethical concerns have to be integrated with concerns for the global. Consequently, for an Arab journalist, Ward might suggest, was to start globalizing his or her practice and participate in the formation of global ethical standards and move away from uncritical forms of patriotism.

Patriotism in Times of Conflict

It is important to note that many Arab journalists have to function and report news in extreme conflict situations. They have to deal with conflict and war stories on both the national and pan-Arab levels. They are frequently reporting either about an inter-state conflict or rivalry between two Arab states as in the cases of Syria–Lebanon, Qatar–Kuwait, and Egypt–Algeria, or in the intra-state conflict, such as the Algerian civil war and the fighting between Hamas and Fatah parties in the Palestinian Territories. In times of conflict and war, a journalist "functions as an active agent in the field" (Liebes and Kampf, 2009, p. 240). Protagonists in conflict attempt to affect the way in which the event is told (Barkho, 2008; Handley, 2009) or framed. Unlike Ward's suggestion, Arab journalists are expected to be patriotic in their coverage of news because the prevalent view among the audiences exists that their countries and region are often attacked, occupied, or threatened. In many ways, Arab journalists seem to be the border guards—if not the architects—of a new imagined Arab *watan* (homeland). Pintak writes,

> They reflect a worldview that largely transcends borders, a sense of self-identity that sets region above nation and religion above passport, and a commitment to political change that is infusing the body politic of the Arab world through the electronic phenomenon of 24/7 news. (2009, p. 193)

In this scenario, Arab journalists have to meet both the expectations of their audiences and avoid upsetting their governments.

In his survey of Arab journalists, Pintak found that Arab journalists' first priority or identification is to their country. Journalists surveyed refer to Arab and Muslim identity as most important with little or no sense of the kind of global journalism Ward has advocated for. Pintak describes Arab journalists as being "decidedly cross-border in their worldview. They have the low sense of identification with their country of citizenship and they are evenly split in terms of identification with the Muslim world versus the Arab region" (Pintak, 2009, p. 196). Valeriani (2010) has proposed the notion of "hybrid transnational space" for Arab journalists as a result of the constant exchanges between the national and pan-Arab news makers. Ramaprasad and Hamdy, in their study of Egyptian journalists, found that "support for Arab values was rated by Egyptian journalists as the most important" and that "support the cause of Palestinians had the highest mean" (2006, p. 176). Fandy has discussed the importance of covering the Palestinian question for Arab journalists in a patriotic manner. He adds that the rationale for this presumed centrality of the Palestinian question for Arab journalists and media is twofold; on the one hand, it is unproblematic and cost-free, meaning it brings no popular or political criticism; on the other hand, it results in higher ratings for the TV station. Ramaprasad and Hamdy emphasize similar arguments in their explanation of the centrality of the support of the cause of the Palestinians among Egyptian journalists. Discussing the Palestinian cause is considered risk-free when compared to investigating and examining the Egyptian government's own policies by Egyptian journalists (Ramaprasad and Hamdy, 2006, p. 181). This can be partially explained by the perceived risk of questioning governmental policies and decisions coupled with audiences' interests in the larger Arab and Muslim *ummah* (community). This same view was expressed by Daud Kattab, who believes that not only pan-Arab channels like Al-Jazeera and Al-Arabiya cover regional issues including the Palestinian–Israeli conflict, Iraq and Lebanon, but local channels follow the same path to escape discussing more controversial issues (Pintak, 2009). What follows are two case-studies which highlight the difficulties of reporting impartially and objectively in the Arab region and ones which show the omnipresence of patriotism in Arab journalism.

Egypt–Algeria Football Match

The clashes between Algerian and Egyptian fans, governments, and media over the World Cup qualifying football match on November 18, 2009, held in Omdurman, Sudan, was called alternately as the "soccer war" and "match of hatred" (Ghazi, 2009). In the aftermath of the match, where Algeria beat Egypt, computer hackers from both countries attacked the other country's newspaper websites (Mayton, 2009). During the clashes, Egyptian media reported about "Algerian terrorism" and Algerians were called "savage barbarians" (Ezz Al-Arab, 2009). The Algerian national liberation movement turned from "a revolution of a million martyrs" into "a nation of a million whores". Similarly, Algerian media began reporting of Egypt as an active collaborator with the United States and Israel against the Palestinians and the killing of innocent Palestinians as well (Ezz Al-Arab, 2009). Mukkaled (2009) wrote for *Al-Sharq Al-Awsat*, the London-based Saudi newspaper, about the role of both Egyptian and Algerian media in instigating hatred between the countries over the football match. She affirms:

> Everybody has had their say on this "war" including the politicians, the athletes, and those in the entertainment industry. However the real stars of this carnival of hatred and those who incited this public anger, unfortunately, are members of the press and media. Well-known journalists and media figures [in both countries] stooped to the level of uttering obscenities and insults; insulting the history, language, and culture of the other country. Fervor and fanaticism have flared up in both countries and there is no sign that this will be contained in the near future ... (Mukkaled, 2009)

Al-Masry Al-Youm was one of the Egyptian newspapers which critically looked at the role of the media in actively instigating hatred towards the Algerians. Egyptian journalists seemed to share the same patriotic rhetoric as the audiences and, often times, instigating a rabid form of patriotism. In this war of words, many Egyptian journalists harshly criticized their own colleagues at *October*, a social and political weekly magazine, for showing the Algerian flag on its cover along with the phrase, "Congratulations Algeria". Many journalists burned copies of the magazine in the streets and called the magazine editors "traitors" (Amer, 2009). Egyptian journalists fell short of voicing any criticism against their own national football team (Nasrawi, 2009). The *Guardian* newspaper indicated that this clash was a diversion of the Egyptians' attention from their frustration towards their own political situation and was instigated by the Egyptian government. The *Guardian*'s piece on these clashes read, "Mubarak [the Egyptian president] and the ruling party took the opportunity to enrage a segment of society that has long been excluded from any political or social advancement. It was a chance to create anger against the 'other' (in this case, Algerians) for what may or may not have occurred" (Shenker, 2009).

In their coverage of the events, Egyptian mainstream media displayed a high level of antagonism towards the Algerian football team and blind support for their own. This was done in the name of the love of Egypt and love for their own country. Many of the mainstream Egyptian media reported alleged deaths of Egyptians attending the November 2009 match in Sudan. This was later denied by the Egyptian foreign ministry (Al-Jazeera, 2009). Global journalism ethics and principles of objectivity, impartiality, and fairness do not seem to have been respected by Egyptian journalists in this case. Many of the Egyptian and Algerian journalists are reported to have exercised high levels of alignment with and advocacy of their respective national soccer team. The Egyptian publication *October* and its journalists were criticized and humiliated for not showing anger and antagonism to the Algerian team, and labeled as unpatriotic.

Arab Journalists and the War on Gaza

In journalism, ethical practices are most important during times of conflict, when national interest of the journalist's own country appears to be at risk. Although, many Arab journalists are inspired by "Anglo-American journalistic practices" (Mellor, 2009, p. 318), many of them believe that these same journalistic ethics have not been very effective in providing news on the Palestinian–Israeli conflict. In other words, ethics of impartiality and objectivity have not guaranteed evenhanded portrayals of the conflict.

The intensive coverage by Al-Jazeera of the second Palestinian Intifada (uprising) 2000 is significant to discuss as it led to Al-Jazeera's establishment as a credible news source in the region (Rugh, 2004). The comprehensive coverage of the intifada made its coverage more attractive for Arab audiences. As of 2008, the Palestinian situation garners the most attention from Arab audiences (Zogby, 2008). Al-Jazeera "reporters and camera crews provided live news and graphic images that were more comprehensive because their news programs were much longer . . . [in doing so] Al-Jazeera established itself as the best Arab news source on Israel and Palestine" (Rugh, 2004, pp. 329–30).

Prior to Al-Jazeera, the coverage of the Palestinian–Israeli conflict had been presented in a biased manner, either towards Israel (by Western news sources) or the Palestinians (by Arab media). Amira Haas, a prominent Israeli journalist and commentator for *Ha'artz*, was asked about one thing that she wants the American media to be doing, she answered, "To stop being afraid of covering what the Israeli occupation and the Israeli regime is doing" (Szremski, 2010). Likewise, Romani (2009) postulates that American journalism has not been successful in safeguarding impartiality when it comes to their own coverage of the Palestinian–Israeli conflict. Although Ahmad al Skaikh, editor-in-chief of Al-Jazeera channel, when asked about the professional criteria used for covering the war on Gaza, explained:

> Our aim was not exactly to report facts as they happen ... this time in which internationalmedia would call the victims of war 'collateral damage' gone forever since the birth of Al-Jazeera channel 12 years ago ... I believe that the focus on the human side of the Gaza war was the cause of stopping the war earlier than planned.

Nabeel Al-Khateeb, editor-in chief at Al-Arabyia news channel, is equally critical of Western media in the United States and the United Kingdom coverage of the Palestinian question, yet he disagrees with al Skaikh's views on journalists' professional duties in this regard. Both journalists criticized the "cold way" in use of phrases such as "collateral damage" in the coverage of war by major international news channels such as CNN, BBC and Sky News. "War coverage has to aim for the ending of the war", they concluded (Shaaban, 2009). While many among the Arab leaders and audiences sometimes call Al-Arabiya news channel Al-Ebryah (the Hebrew) as a way of criticizing its coverage, the real value, al Skaikh emphasizes, is not impartiality but to find ways that we can help "end the war". The ethical standards of impartiality and objectivity in journalism do not guarantee fair representation of the underdog, the Palestinians, in having access of telling their stories in the news media (Najjar, 2009) and Al-Jazeera took such a task.

Al-Jazeera has been critiqued by Al-Khateeb as being a channel which simply "satisfies the mob" and "leads a campaign for Hamas" (Pintak, 2009). In other words, to Al-Jazeera stories emphasized merely popular viewpoints and asserted a pan-Arabic nationalism in their coverage of the Palestinian–Israeli and Iraq conflicts. Al-Jazeera journalists have been accused of serving the Western agenda when they have criticized the status quo in many of the Arab countries. In Egypt, questioning the government policies about religious minorities has been viewed as Al-Jazeera collaborating with the United States. In Lebanon, Al-Jazeera's coverage of Hezbullah and the Syrian presence is seen as its alliance with Syria against Lebanon. Abd Al-Wahhab Badrakhan, former editor-in-chief of the London-based Saudi newspaper *Al-Hayat*, argues that the political challenge that Arab media have to deal with in their journalistic practices shares much in common with others in the world including the United States and Europe (Muhammad, 2010). As Al-Jazeera has shown, Arab journalists have to develop their own ways of covering the Palestinian question. Such coverage may or may not fit with the ideals of impartiality and objectivity as promoted in global journalism scholarship. However, for many of them it is still ethical and balance in according to their own understanding of these professional ideals.

Conclusion

Discussions on journalism ethics are common among Arab journalists. In a region that is filled with conflicts, wars, and injustices, it is natural to think of journalism as a profession that leads to "public good". Many Arab journalists are aware of the significance of committing to ethics of impartiality and balance, though their judgment of global media coverage of their main news story (the Palestinian question) seems to make them doubt the practicality of these ideals in providing just coverage or in achieving public good.

This paper suggests that Arab journalists indicate a deep appreciation of the value of patriotism especially during conflicts and wars. Although many Arab journalists recognize the significance and value of adopting global ethical journalistic principles such as impartiality and objectivity, they still do not demonstrate full adoption of such values especially in situations where they have to actively defend their own country (in the case of Egyptian journalists in coverage of the football match with Algeria) or the pan-Arab region (the Palestinian cause as in Al-Jazeera's coverage of the War on Gaza). In their ethical practice and professional performance, Arab journalists seem to equate patriotism with "public good" and "justice" as in the case of covering the asymmetrical war between Israel and the Palestinians. Patriotism could be considered an ethical virtue if it means "report[ing] independently and keep[ing] interests of citizens in mind" (Elliott, 2004, p. 29). Patriotism, for many in the Arab context, is a virtue and not a breach of journalism ethics though such blind patriotism also leads to lack of criticism of the current political order (authoritarian governments) and lack of press freedom.

REFERENCES

ACTON, LORD (1972) "Nationality", in: *Essays on Freedom and Power*, Gloucester: Peter Smith, pp. 141–70.

AL-ARIAN, LAILA (2004) "Georgetown Conference Scrutinizes Arab Media", *The Washington Report on Middle East Affairs* 23(10), pp. 56.

AL-BAWABA (2010) "Union of Arab Journalists: Arab journalists suffer the lack of freedom", April, http://www1.albawaba.com/ar/, accessed 26 June 2011.

AL-JAZEERA (2009) "Continuous Repercussions of the Match Between Egypt and Algeria", November, http://aljazeera.net/NR/exeres/F2386581-AB5A-4B46-BCCD1571D7FF2F8F.htm, accessed 26 June 2011.

AMER, PAKINAM (2009) "Patriotism Fever Hits Egyptian TV Channels Thanks to Algeria", *Al-Masry Al-Youm*, November, http://www.masress.com/en/almasryalyoumen/3366, accessed 26 June 2011.

AMIN, HUSSEIN (2001) "Mass Media in the Arab States Between Diversification and Stagnation: an overview", in: Kai Hafez (Ed.), *Mass Media, Politics, and Society in the Middle East*, Cresskill, NJ: Hampton Press, pp. 23–42.

BADRAKHAN, ABDUL WAHAB (2006) "The Impact of Occupation on Media Freedom: the cases of Afghanistan and Iraq", in: Emirates Centre for Strategic Studies (Ed.), *Arab Media in the Information Age*, Abu Dhabi: Emirates Center for Strategic Studies, pp. 425–75.

BARKHO, LEON (2008) "BBC'S Discursive Strategy *vis-à-vis* the Palestinian–Israeli Conflict", *Journalism Studies* 9(2), pp. 278–94.

ELLIOTT, DENI (2004) "Terrorism, Global Journalism and the Myth of the Nation State", *Journal of Mass Media Ethics* 19(1), pp. 29–45.

ERICSON, RICHARD (1988) "How Journalists Visualize Facts", *The Annals of the American Academy of Political and Social Science* 560, pp. 83–95.

FANDY, MAMOUN (2007) *(Un) Civil War of Words: media and politics in the Arab world*, London: Praeger.

GHAZI, JALAL (2009) "Egypt vs. Algeria World Cup Violence Comes from Political Frustrations", New America Media: Eye on Arab Media, 17 November, http://news.newamericamedia. org/news/view_article.html?article_id=9a960f417d230e09a31fcb3b9446c465, accessed 26 June 2011.

HAFEZ, KAI (2002) "Journalism Ethics Revisited: a comparison of ethics codes in Europe, North Africa, the Middle East, and Muslim Asia", *Political Communication* 19(2), pp. 225–50.

HAFEZ, KAI (2005) "Arab Satellite Broadcasting: democracy without political parties?", *Transnational Broadcasting Journal*, http://www.tbsjournal.com/Archives/Fall05/Hafez.html, accessed 26 June 2011.

HANDLEY, ROBERT L. (2009) "The Conflicting Israeli-terrorist Image: managing the Israeli–Palestinian narrative in the *New York Times* and *Washington Post*", *Journalism Practice* 3(3), pp. 251–67.

KATEB, GEORGE (2006) *Patriotism and Other Mistakes*, New Haven, CT: Yale University Press.

LIEBES, TAMAR and KAMPF, ZOHAR (2009) "Performance Journalism: the case of media coverage of war and terror", *Communication Review* 12, pp. 239–49.

MACINTYRE, ALASDAIR (1984) "Is Patriotism a Virtue?", The Lindley Lecture, University of Kansas, Lawrence. Reprinted in: I. Primoratz (Ed.) (2002).

MAYTON, JOSEPH (2009) "It's All Patriotism Ahead of Key Algerian–Egyptian Match", *Bikyamasr*, 18 November, http://bikyamasr.com/wordpress/?p = 5871, accessed 26 June 2011.

MELLOR, NOHA (2005) *The Making of Arab News*, Oxford: Rowman & Littlefield.

MELLOR, NOHA (2009) "Strategies for Autonomy: Arab journalists reflecting on their roles", *Journalism Studies* 10(3), pp. 307–21.

MUHAMMAD, AMER (2010) "Badrakhan: Arab media have the obligation to document Israel's crimes", *Islam Today*, September, http://islamtoday.net/nawafeth/mobile/zview-90-139621.htm, accessed 26 June 2011.

MUKKALED, DIANA (2009) "Football and Hate Wars", *Al-Sharq Al-Awsat*, November, http://www.asharq-e.com/news.asp?section = 2&id = 18956, accessed 26 June 2011.

MURPHY, JAMES, B., WARD, STEPHEN J. A. and DONOVAN, ANIE (2006) "Ethical Ideals in Journalism: civic uplift or telling the truth", *Journal of Mass Media Ethics* 21(4), pp. 322–37.

NAJJAR, ABEER (2009) *Conflict Over Jerusalem: covering the Palestinian–Israeli conflict in the British press*, Germany: VDM Verlag.

NASRAWI, SAIF (2009) "Egypt–Algeria: wagging the dog?", *Al-Masry Al-Youm*, November, http://www.almasryalyoum.com/en/news/egypt-algeria-wagging-dog, accessed 26 June 2011.

NORDENSTRENG, KAARLE (Ed.) (1989) *Journalist: status, rights and responsibility*, Prague: International Organization of Journalists.

PINTAK, LAWRENCE (2009) "Gaza: of media wars and borderless journalism", *Arab Media & Society*7, pp. 193–6, http://www.arabmediasociety.com/topics/index.php?t_article =237, accessed 26 June 2011.

PINTAK, LAWRENCE and GINGES, JEREMY (2009) "Inside the Arab Newsroom: Arab journalists evaluate themselves and the competition", *Journalism Studies* 10(2), pp. 157–77.

PRIMORATZ, IGOR (2009) "Patriotism", in: Edward N. Zalta (Ed.), *The Stanford Encyclopedia of Philosophy*, http://plato.stanford.edu/archives/sum2009/entries/patriotism/, accessed 26 June 2011.

REPORTERS WITHOUT BORDERS (2010) *Press Freedom Index 2010*, http://en.rsf.org/press-freedom-index-2010,1034.html, accessed 26 June 2011.

RAMAPRASAD, JOYTIKA and HAMDY, NAILA (2006) "Functions of Egyptian Journalists: perceived importance and actual performance", *International Communication Gazette* 68(2), pp. 167–85.

ROMANI, REBECCA (2009) "The Hazards of Occupation: documentaries by and about Palestinians and Israelis in the Occupied Territories", *Cineaste* 34(3), pp. 1.

RUGH, WILLIAM A. (2004) *Arab Mass Media: newspapers, radio, and television in Arab Politics*, Westport, CT and New York: Praeger Publishers.

SALAITA, STEVEN (2005) "Ethnic Identity and Imperative Patriotism: Arab Americans before and after 9/11", *College Literature* 32(2), pp. 146–68.

SHAABAN, AHMED (2009) "Role of Arab Media in Gaza War Comes Under Scrutiny", *Khaleej Times*, May, http://www.khaleejtimes.com/darticlen.asp?xfile=data/theuae/2009/May/theuae_May310.xml&section=theuae, accessed 26 June 2011.

SHENKER, JACK (2009) "More to Egypt's Riot than Football: the tribalistic violence that followed the World Cup defeat to Algeria was fuelled by a genuine set of grievances", *The Guardian*, 20 November, http://www.guardian.co.uk/commentisfree/2009/nov/25/egypt-riots-football-world-cupd, accessed 26 June 2011.

SYRIAN HUMAN RIGHTS COMMITTEE (2001) "Releasing Nizar Nayuf", *Justice Online Journal* 1(October), http://www.shrc.org/data/aspx/d7/357.aspx, accessed 26 June 2011.

SZREMSKI, KRISTIN (2010) "Amira Hass (Reluctantly) Accepts Courage in Journalism Award", *Washington Report on Middle East Affairs* 29(1), pp. 56–7.

TAN, KOK-CHOR (2004) *Justice Without Borders: cosmopolitanism, nationalism, and patriotism*, Cambridge: Cambridge University Press.

VALERIANI, AUGUSTO (2010) "Pan-Arab Satellite Television and Arab National Information Systems: journalists' perspectives on a complicated relationship", *Middle East Journal of Culture and Communication* 3, pp. 26–42.

WARD, STEPHEN (2004) *The Invention of Journalism Ethics: the path for objectivity and beyond*, Montreal: McGill-Queen's University Press.

WARD, STEPHEN J. A. (2007) "Utility and Impartiality: being impartial in a partial world", *Journal of Mass Media Ethics* 22(2/3), pp. 151–67.

WARD, STEPHEN J. A. (2010) *Global Journalism Ethics*, Montreal: McGill and Queen's University Press.

ZOGBY, JAME (2008) *What Arabs Think: values, beliefs and concerns*, New York: Zogby International.

THE MORALITY OF JOURNALISM ETHICS
Readings of Al Nursi's theory of God's attributes

Abderrahmane Azzi

This paper examines ethics and morality as studied by Al Nursi, a reformist Muslim scholar accredited with the rise of the current Muslim revival in modern Turkey. The paper examines Al Nursi's macro theory of God's attributes and establishes a concise linguistic and semantic link between a sample of God's attributes and journalism ethics. The paper presents a normative perspective on journalism ethics from the religious-Islamic standpoint and maintains that the field of journalism ethics is further enhanced and transformed when the religious source of morality is brought to bear on ethics and practices.

If you find God, you find everything. (Al Nursi)

Introduction

This paper extends Al Nursi's philosophy of ethics to the realm of journalism studies and mass media. Based on his experiences in Turkey, Al Nursi provides a new interpretation on how God's attributes enlighten human experience and can provide moral meanings to life at personal and socio-historical levels. Al Nursi Badi'uzzaman Said (1873–1960) was one of the major architects of contemporary Islamic thinking in Turkey. His voluminous work, *Rasael Al Nur* (*Messages of Light*), based on the essential truths of the Quran, contains the essence of his reformative thought. Literature that seeks to ground journalism media ethics in the religious remains scarce and does not go further than issue of semantics, even though ethics and religion have been important fields of inquiry, both in the West and the East. Al Nursi's work is significant in two ways: (a) it takes a general macro-level stance which postulates that "everything that exist in the Universe is a reflection of one or more of God's attributes" (Al Hanafi, 1966, p. 9) (known as the 99 plus in Islam). In Hadith (Sayings of the Prophet), "Pray with God's attribute, known and those He only know, etc." (Al Ghazali, 2003, p. 167); and (b) it claims that every component of ethics originates in one or many of God's attributes; even the term ethics (Al Qiam in Arabic) is derived from the same linguistic term of one of God's attributes: Al Qayum.

The link between Al Qiam (ethics) and Al Qayum (God's attribute) is well established at the linguistic and semantic levels. This connection between many of God's attributes and ethics that ought to guide human behavior is probably unique to Arabic language and the language of Quran. Ethics, like virtues (in Arabic Akhlaq) derives from God's attribute, Al Khaleq (The Creator) and truthfulness (Al Sidq) derives from God's attribute Al Saadiq (The Truthful). It is Al Nursi's assumption that the meanings of God's attributes are moral guides and enlighten the Universe including human action. While Al Ghazali, a thirteenth-century Muslim scholar, who sought to harmonize science and religion, has done a rigorous analysis of God's attributes, he did not elaborate on the extent to which God's attributes relate to human or social action. Contemporary writers have added little to Al Ghazali's analysis; Al Nursi's theory stands as a major milestone in the development of this inquiry. While Western moral philosophers, rooted in Judeo-Christian tradition, may have found some similarities in this frame of analysis to their own, the dominant Western academia shied away from the connection between ethics and religion. As Singer states, "There existed throughout the Western tradition a split between ethics and religion," but he adds "In Christian theology, systematic attempts were made to eliminate the possibility of a conflict between ethics and religion" (1996, pp. 159–83). This dichotomy still weighs greatly in the global debate on media ethics with regards to universals and proto-norms or what Christians et al. call "ethics of universal being" (2008, p. 135).

This paper argues that the field of journalism ethics is relatively vague and subject to different cultural interpretations partly because of the exclusion of a discussion about morality which puts ethics at a higher context of meanings. The dominant position in journalism and media practices is to consider ethics part of a business and profession. Journalists, it is argued, face ethical dilemmas on a daily basis. Critical and cultural scholars have often elaborated on how media ethics is influenced by politics of news, media systems, and cultural discrepancies. It is easy to see how Al Jazeera, CNN and BBC construct different symbolic realities and fashion public opinion in different ways, even though they all claim to be guided by similar professional ethics such as objectivity, fairness, precision, etc. Media scholars, guided by their arsenal of cognitive and rational thinking as well as by empirical case studies, have had little impact on media practices given that their contributions are usually regarded as mere theoretical assumptions. As communication technologies proliferate, it would be difficult to manage media and journalism practices without a much broader perspective which puts media practitioners and journalists in touch with a larger reality. The intent of this intellectual endeavor is not to completely depart from the existing knowledge and accumulated experiences in journalism ethics, but to provide what the French call "un autre son de cloche" (another sound of the bell—a different story) which engages in the processes of imagination and idealization in order to promote and enhance our search for ethics of journalism ethics. It is not the purpose of this paper to provide solutions, but to present a set of ideas that open new windows in the search of what Weber calls an "ideal type;" a value-oriented approach which provides better understanding of journalism ethics and can be flexible enough to incorporate journalism realities across a variety of cultural and political settings.

The paper postulates that the source of ethics in Al Nursi's thought is to be found in a higher order: religion. This notion is based on two arguments. The first is that humans, being a creation of the Creator as Islam and other monotheist religions maintain, cannot be the source of meanings (as in meanings of life) in a similar but not comparable way that computers cannot function without the necessary software made up by the engineer (the inventor). Humans do not produce but reflect meanings in their actions (behavior). The second is that religious ethics, with reference to Islam specifically, are in tune with human nature which is by itself a creation of the Creator. The moral aspect of ethics can well inform current journalism practices at the theoretical level. It is up to researchers and journalists to create a meaningful balance between what exists and what ought to exist (ideal type). The paper also assumes that at the world of practical (for example, codes of journalism ethics) may not add much to the field of journalism ethics due to, what Al Nursi would call, human limitation as exemplified by the discussion on "who decided what" and "which value judgment" have some universal appeal. The source of ethics is further examined in the light of Al Nursi's philosophical framework.

Al Nursi's Philosophical Framework

Al Nursi's perspective relates to his personal and somewhat tragic experience in a turbulent period of history that saw World War I, the process of secularization taking place in Turkey, the rise of nationalism and what he regarded then as "the clash of civilizations." In his early writings, he was very critical of the materialist aspect of Western civilization. Later, he avoided such a line of argument, saying that the problems facing the Muslims are within (Nursi, 2005, pp. xxi–xxiii). Al Nursi spent 28 years of his life in prison during which time he gained particular insights into the true meaning of the Quran that he viewed as a reflection of God's attribute: Al Nur (The Light) which illuminates the Universe. In his early life (called the old Al Nursi), he was actively engaged in Turkish political life; he maintained that religion was the major force of social change—as such, he is called a social religious reformer—and argued against government policies of secularization, a belief which led to his trials and imprisonment. Later in life (called the new Al Nursi), he devoted his intellectual life to the moral cause. He was once reported to have said, "I seek refuge with God, the Lord of mankind, from Satan and politics" (Bakir, 2003, p. 216). His internal, isolated, and confined religious experience makes him close to the Sufi tradition in Islam, whereby a person withdraws from his/her immediate environment to seek purity and spiritual attachment with God. However, his Sufism, like Al Ghazali's, is mostly reflective and intellectual. For this, he is sometimes labeled as a "philosopher of religion" (Daghamin, 2002, p. 25). His call for social change through peaceful resistance made his ideas popular in the region. The impact of his work is found among his students who are accredited for collecting and later publishing his major work called *Rasael Al Nur* (Messages of Light) which includes *Al Kalimat*, *Al Lamaat*, and *Choaat*. The unavailability of his work in other languages has limited his access to the West. Yet, he stands as a major figure in contemporary Islamic thought and is regarded as "the father" of the modern Islamic movement in Turkey.

The idea of God's attributes has been present in classical Islamic texts. It is outside the scope of this paper to discuss how intellectual pioneers such as Al Bayhaqi, Ibn Hajar, Ibn Arabi and others have written about God's attributes. A brief explanation comes from Al Ghazali who states that there is a need to recognize both the human limitation and the necessity to ponder on the meaning of God's attributes through "vision and retrospection." He argues that "God did not provide a way to know Him except through the inability to know Him" (Al Ghazali, 2003, p. 19) and adds that "No one knows God except Him" (Al Ghazali, 2003, pp. 48–9). Nonetheless, the more we learn about God's attributes as expressed in the Quran, the more we are able to reflect part of those attributes in our lived reality. As such, God created man in his own image. In Hadith, "God created Adam in his own image" (Daghamin, 2002, p. 25). In Al Nursi's words, one reaches true happiness when he/she is guided by God's virtues. In the Quran, we read "That He may make your conduct whole and sound and forgive you your sins: He that obeys Allah and His Messenger has already attained the highest achievement" [The Quran, Al Ahzab (The Confederates), verse 71] (Yusuf, 1989, pp. 1079–80).

In his understanding of God's attributes, Al Nursi combines both macro and micro analyses of religious texts (the Quran and Hadith, sayings of the Prophet Mohamed). At the macro level, he views the Universe as a coherent system where everything fits together by way of reflecting one or many of God's attributes. He maintains that every verse in the Quran surrounds and encompasses the cosmos in its totality. The "Light" verse is a case in point. The verse describes God as the Light which, in Al Nursi's interpretation, guides everything that exists: Allah is the Light of the heavens and the earth. The parable of His Light is as (if there were) a niche and within it a lamp; the lamp is in a glass, the glass as it were a brilliant star, lit from a blessed tree, an olive, neither of the East nor of the West, whose oil would almost glow forth though no fire touched it. Light upon light! Allah guides to His Light whom He wills. And Allah sets forth parables for mankind, and Allah is All-Knower of everything. At the micro level, he observes the smallest creature (a cell, a flower) in the Universe to explain the meanings of God's attributes as reflected in the behavior of such creatures. In his words, everything starts with God and ends with God. The Quran states that everything that exists prays to God but we only do not understand the languages of such creatures. In the Quran, it is written, "The seven heavens and the earth and all beings therein, declare His glory: There is not a thing but celebrates His praise: and yet ye understand not how they declare His glory! Verily, He is Oft-Forbearing, Most Forgiving!" [the Quran, Al Ahzab (The Confederates), verse 44] (Yusuf, 1989, p. 686).

The disintegration of the Muslim society (Ummah) is not the result of chance or external forces as much as the result of internal processes which pulls away from the main source of strength (the moral base) in favor of gains in the material world. In this, Al Nursi's perspective is similar to such early religious reformers as Al Afghani, leader of the religious reformation movement in the Muslim World in the late nineteenth century and Ibn Badis, leader of the religious reformation movement in Algeria in the 1930s. However, his approach is unique in the way he interprets God's attributes in daily life. In Al Nursi's theory of God's attributes, it is pertinent to distinguish between connected and disconnected ethics. Connected ethics are those concepts that originate in religious texts; they can be traced etymologically to the Quran. Conversely, disconnected ethics are pure rational endeavors without any apparent attachment to a higher order of morality as God's attributes.

Nature and Meaning of God's Attributes

Humans, in projecting God's attributes, hold "real" power; they are empowered by their Creator (Nursi, 2008b, pp. 193—4). Al Nursi states that everything that exists in the Universe obeys the rules of God through the reflection of one or many of His attributes. Thus, a flower which shines with beauty is a sign of God's mastery of creating the best of everything and a reflection of God's attribute, Al Jamil (The Beautiful). In the Quran, we read, "Verily, We created man in the best stature (mold)" (The Quran, At Tin (The Fig), verse 4). Al Nursi writes, "Who has beauty of vision has beauty of thought, and who has beauty of thought finds pleasure in life" (Awis, 2009, p. 164). This principle stands for every province of meaning including, for example, the sphere of knowledge. Human knowledge, even though limited as stated in the Quran, "Of knowledge it is only a little that is communicated to you, O men" [Quran, Al Isra (The Journey by Night), verse 85] (Yusuf, 1989, p. 698), is a projection of God's attribute: Al Alim (The Knower); Law is a projection of

God's attribute: Al Adel (The Fair); Medicine is a projection of God's attribute: Al Shafi (The Healer), among others. To Al Nursi, God, in his attributes, is the highest ideal and the final destination for everything that exist. In his words, everything seeks God and "who finds God finds everything." It would be beyond the scope of this paper to deal with each and every one of God's attributes as described by Al Nursi. For this paper I will discuss six attributes to explain Al Nursi's general approach to God's attributes

God's attributes take a particular significance in Al Nursi's perspective whereby every attribute enlightens every sphere of human action including journalism ethics. Some attributes, for example, include the following.

1. Al Qudous (The Holy)

The Holy refers to the act of neatness. To Al Nursi, "the cleanness, purity, clarity and splendor that we witness in the Universe is the work of The Holy. Without His will, dirt, filth and waste that goes along with the death of hundreds of thousands of different creatures not to mention the rubbish that come with dead leaves, spoiled vegetation and the garbage that humans turn out daily—could have turned the Universe into a messy, fetid, and decaying milieu of high proportion" (Nursi, 2007, p. 465). The Holy also has resonance in God's order that is put into action by insects, bugs, and eagles that play the role of garbage collectors and waste disposals. Even the white cells in our blood are actually echoes of the true meaning of The Holy by the mere act of purifying the human body from germs much like our elbows protect our eyes from dust and alien objects.

2. Al Hakam (The Judge)

Al Nursi states that this attribute infers the highest form of organization and unity without which the Universe would fall into disarray. Every detail in the Universe is accounted for and made to behave in accordance with God's will. The example of a tree may exemplify the nature of the Universe; a tree is a word; its fruits are letters of that word, its seeds are points for the letters, and all reflect a unique glossary of terms and an independent code of behavior in accordance with a higher order of meaning: religion.

3. Al Fard (The One)

The unity of the Universe reflects the Unity of the Creator (the One), and everything in the Universe points to God's oneness (Nursi, 2008b, p. 219). The One is the Cause of everything; He has no need of anyone and everyone is in need of Him. He is not like anyone while everyone is a projection of one or many of His attributes (Nursi, 2007, p. 495).

4. Al Hay (Alive)

Life is a reflection of God's attribute Al Hay (Alive). It is through His Light that the Universe is enlightened. The concept of life (Al Hayat) is privileged because human life continues after death. It is the spiritual dimension that keeps life alive. To live for the sake of worldly life (here and now) defeats the purpose of existence. To Al Nursi, the wisdom of creation is to project God's attributes; when a thing accomplishes the mission of such a projection, it ceases to exist and leaves the way for newer beings. The Universe is like a blackboard and God writes and erases things in accordance with His Words.

5. Al Qayu (The Ethical)

The entire enterprise of ethics is a reflection of God's attributes (The Ethics). Everything that exists does so because of Him (The Care Taker). In Arabic language, it is linguistically unfeasible to disassociate ethics from The Ethical. The uniqueness of Arabic is very informative and striking in the sense that the etymology of Arabic concepts of ethics leads to God's attributes. Unfortunately, not much scholarly work has been done about the aspects of Al Qayum as God's attributes and the existing journalism ethics literature in the Middle East mostly replicates Western perspectives.

Journalism Ethics Literature and the Profession of Journalism

The contemporary philosophy of media and journalism ethics do not surpass core ideas found in the enlightenment treaties such as those in John Stuart Mill's "On Liberty" (Mill, 1947). The social responsibility theory of media sought to overcome inherent shortcomings of the libertarian framework, but the theory did not achieve much beyond the level of harnessing certain awareness among media professionals. In Al Nursi's theory, it would be difficult to talk about ethics outside the realm of religion (God's attributes). Most current journalism ethics are the product of Western experience. Still, one should not exclude the religious component in such ethics if we assume that, as Weber has documented, there is a relationship between "protestant ethics and the spirit of capitalism." There has been a trend among academics in media and journalism studies to reduce media ethics to codes of ethics which, even though informative and constructive, have little power to influence the professional practice of journalists. This is the case especially in the Arab/Islamic setting. These codes, including the ones in the Middle East, have a "libertarian" inclination in which the theoretical grounds of such ethics relate to the philosophy of enlightenment, and incorporate little about Islamic ideals. Ethical decision making is left to individuals, to different institutional and cultural conditions, and to circumstances. Since the introduction of the "Canons of Journalism" by the American Society of Newspaper Editors in 1923, the concepts of objectivity, liberty, fairness, separation of facts from opinions, honesty, truthfulness, comprehensiveness, neutrality, respect of privacy, independence, responsibility, seriousness and decency echoed almost everywhere. The separation of facts from opinions, in particular, is well emphasized in US media. In the Arab/Islamic setting, those notions are appealing but the media reality is far from such journalistic traditions. These canons achieved universality based on the facile belief that "what is good for the West is 'probably' good for everyone else." There are few cross-cultural analyses of the subject. In his attempt to make the case for the universality of certain ethics, Deni Elliot presented the view of certain philosophers who argue, for example, that death and handicaps are evils in all cultures. While grief at losing someone as a family member may exist in any culture, the way death or sickness is perceived and experienced varies from one cultural context to another. In Islam, and presumably in other monotheist religions, death is part of the truth of existence and a test to measure the degree to which an individual believes in God's will. The more the individual shows patience, the more he/she is rewarded thereafter. It would be wrong to assume that people everywhere have similar perceptions and understanding of such concepts (Elliot, 1997). The intellectual discussion of journalism ethics in Arab and Muslim societies was always limited and most media institutions adapted ethics terminology from the West to present themselves as modern.

Al Nursi's Perspective and Journalism Ethics

The intellectual history of media ethics in the Arab and Muslim societies is limited. A critical review (Azzi, 2005) of codes of ethics in the Arab region beginning with the Chapter of the Federation of Arab Journalists (FAJ) in 1970 to the newly adapted Al Jazeera's Code of Ethics in 2004 shows that there exists a disparity in the narrative make-up of codes of ethics from one country to another. The entity which issues such codes is mostly an official or semi-official authority (Ministry of Information, Association of Journalists and other government or semi-independent media institutions). There also exists ambiguity in cultural and ideological references in these codes; a number of the codes take an authoritarian stance; some have a pan-Arab nationalist orientation and others have a more liberal bent (i.e., Al Jazeera). Such codes have evolved in many directions throughout the region. There are three major themes that can be paraphrased as constituting the contents of such codes: (1) the first is an effort to promote professional aspect of journalism; (2) the second is that the journalist is theoretically accountable to the government, the public, and works to promote abstract concepts such as nation, national interests, national security, etc., and (3) journalists have restrictions such as restrictions in criticizing officials (especially the President or the King). What these codes do not give us are ideals or value systems. As I have discussed earlier, Al Nursi's theory can enrich these codes and the intellectual discussions of media ethics in the Middle East by giving a morally based vision of ethics and a moral guide for the journalist in his or her capacity as "transmitter of truth."

Given the brevity of space, it is impossible to discuss Al Nursi's discussion of all known God's attributes (99 plus). I discuss below six of God's attributes and how each might enrich our discussions in journalism ethics and the professional practices of journalists. Each of these attributes, I suggest, can impact the way journalists perceive and approach their profession. The underlying meaning of "communication" is significant in that regards given that the Books (the Bible, the Talmud, and the Quran) are communication between God and Man. The first revealed verse in the Quran begins with the verb, Read, "Proclaim (or Read): In the name of thy Lord and Cherisher, Who created—created man, out of a (mere) clot of congealed blood: Proclaim and thy Lord is most Bountiful—He Who taught (the use of) the pen—Taught man that which he knew not" [the Quran, Surat Al-Alaq (The Clot), verses 1–5] (Yusuf, 1989, pp. 1672–3). The six of God's attributes which Al Nursi discusses and which might help us to understand larger issues of morality as they relate to journalism ethics are as follows.

Al Moamin (The Faithful)

It is one of the main traits of the communicator to have faith (religious faith) without which his or her ethical stance is left to his or her individual and idiosyncratic judgment, to the news organization and cultural makeup of society, all of which involve human limitations. Al Nursi states that, "The highest purpose of man and the essence of human nature is the belief in God; the highest position of knowledge is to know God; the utmost happiness and gift for man and angels is to love God; and the best and pure reward for man is the spiritual satisfaction." The sphere of journalism, with its major impact on the public, is too important to be left in the hands of a mere journalist or of a single media organization with little understanding of morality. While the individual journalist is free not to believe, he or she must enter a new space with a sense of social and moral responsibility in line with Al Nursi's perspective. The issues of depiction of violence, libel, invasion of privacy, etc., would not arise if Al Moamin was a major tenet among journalists.

Al Haaq (The Reality)

The role of the communicator is also to constantly search for "reality." The concept of "reality" is controversial at many levels; what is real for an individual or a society may not be the case for another individual or society. The sociology of knowledge has provided an elaborate theoretical framework in which the concept of "reality" is called into question. The theory argues that "reality is socially constructed" (Berger, 1967). In line with the same argument, a number of cultural theorists have suggested that "reality is media constructed." These interpretations would not support Al Nursi's theory that reality is a reflection of God's attribute (The Real); it is that action (individual, social or historical) which mirrors attributes and leads to God. He states, "Everything begins with God and ends with God." As such, journalism practices ought to be measured by the degree to which they project ideals of morality and God's attributes. When God is "present" and brought to action, the journalist enters the realm of morality at individual, institutional and historical levels. In Al Nursi's words, man wonders around reality and it is his Al Ghafla (lapses) that deviates him from the right path.

Al Adel (The Fair)

The complexity of the Universe requires a precise balance that keeps everything in a state of unity with everything else. This process can only be directed by God in his attribute as The Fair. Al Adel is the inspiration for justice as reflected in the need for social justice, the justice for those who hold different opinions and justice for wrongdoers (Al Khatib, 2009, p. 12). In the Quran, we read that Muslims must live the middle way. The role of the journalists involves the ability to balance facts and opinions given that life, i.e., political life, is a complex process that involves good and evil. It is through the act of balance (Al Ade) that good prevails over evil. This process is called tadafoa (pushing one another to the right direction) and against clash or conflict.

Al Saadiq (The Truthful)

Truthfulness means "telling the truth" to the best of one's ability as a journalist. In Al Nursi's perspective, truthfulness is moral in nature. Deciding what course of action to follow, which news story to cover, what policy to adapt, whether to wage a war or seek peace is a moral stance. Truthfulness includes getting things right as far as facts and opinions are concerned. It is part of truthfulness to base arguments and policies on real information. It also involves the process by which one's action corresponds to one's ethics; that is, telling the truth not with a non-concerned detached posture but as a conscious endeavor that springs from a deeper moral stance. Al Nursi maintains that one major factor which accounts for the state of decadence in Muslim communities is the absence of Al Saadiq (Omar, 1997, p. 61) in social and political life. While journalists, especially in the West, value the notion of truthfulness through a number of "disconnected" ethics such as objectivity, sincerity, etc., they are, like media elsewhere, constantly subject to manipulation of all sorts. Chomsky has well documented how the US media manufactures public consent to justify certain political policies of the ruling government in Latin America and Asia (Chomsky, 1988). Similarly, an influential political figure in the United States has made the case that the whole enterprise of invading Iraq in 2004 was based on what he calls "convenient untruths" (Gore, 2007, pp. 100–28). It is problematic how the US media, with its history of journalistic traditions and claims of freedom, fairness and neutrality, was not able to resist such "convenient untruths" and missed "inconvenient truths" in a major conflict with severe political ramifications.

Al Hakam (The Judge)

In Al Nursi's theory, man is the index and glossary (Fahras) (Nursi, 2008a, p. 29) of the Universe. He incorporates the manifestation of God's attributes. In the Quran, we read, "We have honoured the sons of Adam; provided them with transport on land and sea; given them for sustenance things good and pure; and conferred on them special favours; above a great part of Our creation" [the Quran, Al Isra (The Journey by Night), verse 70] (Yusuf, 1989, p. 694). While being part of the community wins over the notion of isolation or individualism, man is distinguished from other creatures by his ability to think and make decision on his own which he calls "the relative I." After all, the individual will be judged thereafter as such. Independence is not from but within the enterprise of morality. It involves the ability to refrain from blind adherence to clannish or ideological beliefs. The position of the journalist, as an independent actor "from within," is critical in society. Human beings are full of contradictions that can only be understood by an independent and enlightened mind. This notion is more than independence from governments, market interests, etc.; it is a moral independence which resists unquestioned assumptions.

Al Hasib (The Accountant)

Al Nursi argues that an individual ought to constantly engage in self-reflection and examine his action in light of a higher value system. In a well-known prose, Umar bin Al Khattab, the Second Muslim Caliph, states, "Make yourself accountable before you are made accountable (by God)" (Al Ghazali, 2008, p. 1872). The journalist who works in the public domain is to be held more accountable than others. In the Quran, we read, "Not a word does he utter but there is a sentinel by him, ready (to note it)" [the Quran, Qaf, verse 18] (Yusuf, 1989, p. 1349). The media do little self-examination or self-criticism; they tend to assume they are "right." In Al Nursi's theory, accountability is dictated by moral considerations. As media evolves in an ever-changing social and technological environment, journalists are subjected to ethical challenges which can only and effectively be addressed through, Al Hasib, or self-reflective moral examination. The above-mentioned attributes give us examples of how Al Nursi's theory connects human behavior (and media practices) to the highest ideal of God's attributes.

Conclusion

In this paper, it was argued that Al Nursi's theory could be instructive for journalists and scholars in media ethics. Al Nursi puts morality at the center of any ethical endeavor and opens possibilities for further intellectual exploration. His theory questions current scholarly and academic trends in media ethics, especially in the Arab Muslim context, given that most codes of ethics in the region lack reference to a higher system of values. Al Nursi's theory calls on journalists and media professionals to ponder on God's attributes in their everyday business. This is more than inviting man to faith or to be "a good citizen." It goes beyond the realm of "traditional morality" to provide a concise account of how God's attributes relate to human action and the Universe. The paper sought to relate Al Nursi's theory of ethics in a selective manner; the way a number of God's attributes can shape the intellectual and philosophical inquiries in media and that every concept of journalism ethics is a reflection of one of God's attributes. Future studies could contemplate on many other of God's attributes (known as 99+). No doubt that it takes the knowledge and the spiritual experience of an Al Ghazali, St Augustine, Buddha, and Al Nursi to engage in such an extremely difficult field of inquiry. In Al Nursi's works we find a new understanding of morality whose source is in religion and a particular vision of God's attributes which could inspire journalists and those in the media profession.

REFERENCES

AL GHAZALI, ABU HAMED (2003) *Al Maksid Al Asna fi Sharh Maani Asma Allahi Al Husna* [*The Highest Purpose in Explaining the Meanings of God's Attributes*], Bassam Abud Wahab Al Ghabi (Ed.), Beirut: Dar Ibn Hazm.

AL GHAZALI, ABU HAMED (2008) *Ihya Olum el Din* [*Revival of Religious Sciences*], Beirut: Dal Al Fikr Al Arabi.

AL HANAFI, ABULMUNAIM (1966) *Tajaliat fi Asma Allahi al Husna* [*Echoes in God's Attributes*], Cairo: Maktabat Madbouli.

AL KHATIB, ABDULLAH (2009) "Athar Rasael al Nur fi Nachr al Adala al Fardiya wel Ijtimaia" ["The Impact of Rasael al Nur 'Messages of Light' on the Diffusion of Individual and Social Justice"], unpublished research paper, University of Sharjah, United Arab Emirates.

AWIS, ABDELHAMID (2009) *Rajolo al Qura'n wa Sinaato al Insan* [*The Man of the Quran and the Transformation of Man*], Istanbul: Dal Al Nil.

AZZI, ABDERRAHMANE (2005) "Code of Ethics in the Arab Region: a critical evaluation", paper presented to the Media Ethics Conference, United Arab Emirates University, December.

BAKIR, HASSAN ABDULRAHMAN (2003) *Nursi, Bediuzzaman Said wa Atharoho fi al Fikr wal Daawa* [*Nursi, Bediuzzaman Said and His Impact on Thought and Propagation of Faith*]. Electronic book, http://aljsad.net/showthread.php?t=140518.

BERGER, PETER (1967) *The Social Construction of Reality: a treatise in the sociology of knowledge*, New York: Anchor Books.

CHOMSKY, NOAM (1988) *Manufacturing Consent: The Political Economy of the Mass Media*, New York: Pantheon.

CHRISTIANS, CLIFFORD, RAO, SHAKUNTALA, WARD, STEPHEN J. A. and WASSERMAN, HERMAN (2008) "Toward a Global Media Ethics: theoretical perspectives", *Ecquid Novi: African Journalism Studies* 29(2), pp. 135–72, http://ajs.uwpress.org/cgi/content/refs/29/2/135, accessed 12 October 2010.

DAGHAMIN, ZIYAD (2002) "Mathahir Tkrim al Insan fi al Bayan al Qurani: Qiraa fi Fikr Al Nursi" ["Facets of Honoring Man in the Quran: Readings in Al Nursi's Thought"], *Dirasat* [*Studies Journal*], 29, 39–56.

ELLIOT, DENI (1997) "Universal Values and Moral Development Theories", in: Clifford Christians and Michael Traber (Eds), *Communication Ethics and Universal Values*, London: Sage, pp. 68–82.

GORE, AL (2007) *The Assault on Reason*, New York: The Penguin Press.

MILL, JOHN STUART (1947) *On Liberty,* Alburey Castell (Ed.), Northbrook, Illinois.

NURSI, BEDIUZZAMAN SAID (2005) *The Words: the reconstruction of Islamic belief and thought*, Huseyin Alkarsu (Trans.), Somerset, New Jersey: Light.

NURSI, BEDIUZZAMAN SAID (2007) *Al Lamaat* [*Sparks*], Ihsan Kacem Al Salhi (Trans.), Istanbul: Dar al Nil.

NURSI, BEDIUZZAMAN SAID (2008a) *Sayra Thatia; Kulliyat Rasael El Nur* [*Autobiography*], Ihsan Kacem Al Salhi (Trans.), Istanbul: Dar al Nil.

NURSI, BEDIUZZAMAN SAID (2008b) *Al Kalimat* [*Words*], Ihsan Kacem Al Salhi (Trans.), Istanbul: Dar al Nil.

OMAR, AHMED MOKHTAR (1997) *Asma Allah Al Husan: Dirasa fi al Binya wa al Dilaly* [*God's Attribute: a study in structure and meanings*], Cairo: Alam Al Koutoub.

SINGER, IRVING (1996) *The Harmony of Nature and Spirit*, Baltimore, MD: The Johns Hopkins University Press.

YUSUF, ALI ABDULLAH (1989) *The Meaning of the Holy Quran*, Beltsville, MD: Amana Publications.

TELEVISION REALITY SHOWS IN THE ARAB WORLD
The case for a "glocalized" media ethics

Muhammad Ayish

As much as Western-style reality television in the Middle East has gained extensive popularity among the region's audiences, it has also provoked serious ethical questions. In addressing this emerging genre, some television channels have evolved their own reality shows that emphasize local values and traditions. Based on a survey study and a focus group discussion involving University of Sharjah (United Arab Emirates) students who were exposed to two sets of reality shows, one "globalized" and the other "localized", it was clear that both were perceived to carry converging and diverging universal and Arab-Islamic values and norms. The findings of the study suggest that convergence between indigenous and universal media ethics supports the case for a "glocalized" media ethics the Arab world needs to sustain its emerging media industries in a global context.

Introduction

Recent transitions in the Arab communications landscape as marked by satellite broadcasting have not only induced the proliferation of hundreds of television channels, but have also given rise to imported global programs genres, the most controversial of which is reality television. According to the market consultancy firm, Arab Advisors Group (2008), reality television formats in the Arab world emerged after the introduction of the 2003 *Superstar* show on Lebanese Future TV, followed by the Lebanese Broadcasting Corporation's (LBC) *Star Academy*. Ever since, the region's television sphere has served as a launching pad for scores of Western-style reality television shows like *Big Brother*, *Fear Factor*, *Ton of Gold*, *Perfect Bride*, *The Chef Star*, and *Mission Fashion*. In its 2010 survey of reality television markets in the Middle East, Arab Advisors Group (2010) noted that reality shows are spurred by media market liberalization, and a boom in satellite television and viewership.

But while reality television has been hailed as a success story among private broadcasters, advertisers, and producers, it has not always been perceived as such by the region's publics. This genre's reflection of "candid" living experiences, especially those involving open and intimate male–female relations, and its focus on specific issues widely perceived to have "the least redeeming moral and social values", were bound to keep itself at the center of political and cultural controversies. In early 2008, Arab information ministers issued a "Satellite Television Charter" calling for the restriction of television content with "damaging cultural and social effects" (Amin, 2008). In October 2009, leaders of the six-member Gulf Cooperation Council adopted a declaration addressing adverse television effects on children and the youth (Doha Declaration, 2008). Across the region,

Future Television's *Super Star*, LBC's *Star Academy*, and MBC's *Big Brother* shows have provoked critical reactions. It is often argued that these shows were encroaching on cultural values and traditions through their featuring of unfettered male—female relations (Ayish, 2008). In 2006, hundreds of people took to the streets in Bahrain to protest MBC's planned taping of a *Big Brother*-style show in which young men and women were supposed to be living together under the same roof.

The region's reactions to Western-style reality television have not been confined to public complaints and official condemnations. Broadcasters themselves have shown aversion to those formats by evolving their own reality shows that lend themselves more to the region's peculiar cultural traditions. It is widely believed that as a genre, reality television has a huge potential for shaping public opinion on wide-ranging social and cultural issues as long as it functions within the parameters of Arab-Islamic morality. When properly harnessed, this format can even be instrumental for promoting democracy in the region (Ayish, 2009; Kraidy, 2007). Based on these assumptions, culturally "localized" reality television seems to have emerged as a response to "globalized" reality shows that draw on Western-style social and moral values. Examples include shows like Abu Dhabi Channel's *Million's Poet*, Qatar Television's *Stars of Science*, and Dubai Television's *Innovators*. Localized programs primarily endeavor to promote specific values relating to religious morality, eloquence, and scientific creativity.

This article addresses how both "globalized" and "localized" reality shows are perceived by youthful publics in the region. Based on a survey and a focus-group discussion involving University of Sharjah (United Arab Emirates) students who were exposed to three episodes of two "localized" and two "globalized" Arabic reality shows, the study explores how both sets of programs were rated against a set of cultural and moral values. The "globalized" shows include: LBC's *Star Academy* and Future Television's *Super Star*, while the "localized" ones include Abu Dhabi Channel's *Million's Poet* and Qatar Television's *Stars of Science*. It should be noted here that both reality show categories are not taken as epitomizing two mutually-exclusive cultural values, but do share significant features that could support the case for a "glocalized" media ethics in the region.

Television Ethics in the Middle East: The Ongoing Debate

In a region immersed in serious ferment, the introduction of Western-style formats and contents was bound to create heated political, cultural and ethical debates. Across the Arab world, most television organizations were inclined to develop codes of ethics that stress professional values like accuracy, objectivity, impartiality, responsibility, balance, and freedom. The most outstanding code of ethics has been evolved by al Jazeera satellite channel. al Jazeera's code stresses adherence "to the journalistic values of honesty, courage, fairness, balance, independence, credibility and diversity, giving no priority to commercial or political considerations over professional ones" (al Jazeera, 2008). al Jazeera's rival, al Arabiya, has created its own code of ethics lending itself more to international than to local professional standards. In the UAE, Dubai Media Inc., Abu Dhabi TwoFour54 Media Authority, Dubai Media City, and Sharjah Television have their own codes of ethics that draw on both local and global professional orientations and norms. In 2009, the UAE Journalists' Association joined hands with the International Federation of Journalists (IFJ) in launching an "ethical media initiative" (IFJ, 2010). The initiative is described as "a non-binding and voluntary program that will attempt to regulate journalistic practices in areas of accountability, ethics, equality and objectivity" (IFJ, 2010).

An important feature of the Arab world's media ethics movement is its emphasis on indigenous morality. Advocates of relativist ethical standards in this region often invoke the peculiar social, political, and cultural contexts in which media institutions operate to argue against globalized visions. Arab societies in the Middle East and North Africa, generally conservative in their lifestyles and values, are dominated by patriarchal political and social traditions that would always impact on how media operate. Prevailing tribal and religious orientations normally militate against the institution of Western-style media systems founded on freedom of speech and adversarial state relationships. In state-controlled media institutions, issues of national interest, as defined by the state, are of paramount importance in legal and ethical regulatory schemes. Religious and inherited cultural traditions relating to expression, gender, morality, the individual, and the community have been instrumental in defining how media handle sensitive social and political issues (Ayish and Badawi, 1997).

But the growing globalization of communications industries in the Middle East seems to have given rise to a new brand of professional ethics that preserves fundamental indigenous morality, without alienating global standards. Growing Arab publics' exposure to international media through satellite television and the Web seems to have enhanced their appreciation of how television content needs to be handled, at least in technical terms. The notion of filming people in real-life situations doing something innovative with redeeming moral and social values has never been stranger to the region's publics. For over six decades, television broadcasting has been entrusted with a major "developmental function" that would be conveniently carried out through innovative formats like reality shows. Hence, the notion of "localization" or "indigenization" has come to gain much vogue in recent years as local broadcasters sought to accommodate local moral values and globalized television standards. It is true that television is a Western invention; yet, as the sample student population surveyed in this study noted, it can be harnessed to promote indigenous social and cultural traditions. What matters here is not the medium *per se*, but how it is used in the context of well-defined ethical standards.

There is, however, no consensus in the Arab region that all Western-style television reality shows are ethically subversive. The growing popularity of LBC's *Star Academy* and Future Television's *Super Star* suggest how divided the region has been along social and cultural lines when it comes to how individuals, especially the youth, identify themselves. In one of the rare, yet most exciting scholarly works on reality television in the Middle East, Kraidy (2009) reveals the pull between traditional cultural values and the modernization of Arab society, and the ways in which reality television in the Islamic world is communicating the ideas behind modern beliefs. Kraidy provides specific examples that highlight how different groups have used the medium of reality television to further their agenda and how popular culture can become political currency. In another study on public perceptions of reality TV shows, al Kaaki (2008) noted how this format is providing young women and men with alternative entertainment that offsets the heavy dose of political talk shows carried by channels like al Jazeera and al Arabiya. It has also been argued that reality shows offer individuals opportunities for public participation and expression that they normally would not find in their own communities (Kraidy, 2005).

Debates on Global Media Ethics

Ward defines global journalism ethics as aiming at "developing a comprehensive set of principles and standards for the practice of journalism in an age of global news media" (2005, p. 4). Though the notion of "glocalization" or "hybridization" of media ethics has enjoyed a good amount of scholarly currency, it was in the post-9/11 era that the issue received substantive attention. In 2003, a special issue of the *Journal of Media Ethics* discussed ideas on whether there can be a universal set of moral values toward which media professionals may look for guidance. Contributors saw the September 11 attacks as creating the need for a commitment to global communitarianism to align powerful Western media and the rest of the world. Long before 9/11, however, Christians had spearheaded a remarkable intellectual drive for a global media ethics rooted in what he termed "universal proto-norms" shared by human cultures (Christians and Traber, 1997). Cognizant of the fact that theoretical debates about global media ethics are marked by disagreements about the nature, possibility, and desirability of a global ethics, Christians et al. (2008) champion what they label as an "ethics of universal being" expressed by such universals as the sacredness of life, truth, and nonviolence. According to Steiner (2011), the compelling ethical legacy of Christians and his profound commitment to moral action is enriched by his engagement with universal "proto-norms", values that order all human relationships and institutions and so bypass the divisiveness of appeals to individual rights, cultural practices, or national prerogatives.

For some scholars, the construction of a global media ethics is a natural response to increasing media globalization. Ward (2008) refers to the emergence of a global media ethics movement comprising scholars, global-minded journalists, websites and international journalism associations who are united in their belief that the globalization of news media requires a re-thinking of the principles of journalism. As the "public" of journalism turns increasingly trans-national, basic norms, such as objectivity, should be interpreted from an international perspective. In answering the question of why journalism ethics should go global, Ward (2008) argues that in a radically connected world, news media should report on events in a way reflecting a global plurality of views. It should practice a journalism that helps different groups understand each other, and avoid conflict. Among other things, Ward (2008) notes that a global journalism ethics reins in parochial media inclinations such as extreme patriotism. He cites the case of how some news organizations during the Iraq War of 2003 so quickly shucked their peacetime commitments to independent, impartial reporting as soon as the drums of war started beating.

The genesis of global media ethics goes back to the early 1990s as tensions between the local and the global came to dominate academic and policy discussions of media development, especially in developing nations. According to Robertson (1995, p. 26), who is credited with popularizing the term, "glocalization" describes "the compression of the world and the intensification of the consciousness of the world as a whole". Though Robertson's notion of "glocalization" has received ample criticism from researchers, it has remained a defining framework for understanding how the local relates to the global in different disciplines, including media ethics. Rao and Wasserman (2007), for example, sought ways to integrate "local" or "indigenous epistemologies" within global media ethics. In a comparative study of media ethics among journalists in India and South Africa, Wasserman and Rao (2008) found a two-way relationship between global and local epistemologies and practices. They suggested a global-to-local theoretical matrix that takes into consideration the complexity of journalism ethics in specific cultural and national contexts. Tehranian (2002) takes peace as a central universal value on which sustainable media ethics could be founded. He argues that in a globalized world, media ethics must be negotiated not only professionally but also institutionally, nationally, and internationally.

In the Middle East, the advent of satellite television and the World Wide Web has offered unique opportunities for local and global media to converge. Though debates on this issue have failed to generate any genuine region-specific media ethics perspectives, the adoption of global program formats and genres to communicate with local audiences across the region was bound to foster interest in this field.

Method

The study draws on a January 2010 survey of an 80-student sample from the University of Sharjah who were exposed to three episodes of two sets of reality television shows representing "globalized" and "localized" formats. The globalized was represented by LBC's *Star Academy* and Future Television's *Super Star* and the localized represented by Abu Dhabi Channel's *Million's Poet* and Qatar Television's *Stars of Science* shows. The survey findings were supplemented with the results of a focus-group discussion carried out on April 15, 2010 and involving 20 students who participated in the survey. Students were asked to rate their perception of the strength of each one of the following 10 social and moral values assumed to be carried by the shows on a five-point scale: (1) Freedom, (2) Responsibility, (3) Decency, (4) Intimacy, (5) Individualism, (6) Innovation, (7) Diversity, (8) Honor, (9) Participation, and (10) Cooperation. In the context of the ongoing debate in the region about the ethical implications of satellite television on cultural traditions and values, the survey seeks to find out how television publics in the Arab world perceive television-mediated morality through reality shows.

An Overview of the Four Reality Shows

Super Star (Future Television; year of launch: 2003). Launched by Lebanese Future Television, *Super Star* was believed to have enhanced Future Television's stature both nationally and regionally as thousands of Arabs auditioned to participate in the program and millions watched and voted for their favorite contestants (Kraidy, 2005). The show draws on having three contestants perform on stage in front of jurors. Both young men and women from different Arab countries, in Western-style dresses, sought to impress the in-studio jury and audience as well as the wider publics across the Middle East with their singing performance. But as Kraidy (2005) notes, as the show reached its final weeks, it turned from an artistic competition between individual contestants to an international rivalry in which each contender was primarily performing as a representative of their country. The show is performed in highly glamorous musical atmospheres reflecting a clearly liberal outlook. In its premier appearance in summer 2003, the show was instrumental in polarizing audiences on patriotic and nationalistic grounds.

Star Academy (LBC Television; year of launch: 2003). Star Academy has been considered the most controversial reality television show in the region. It draws on playing host to young men and women serving as performing arts students who aspire to be stars in their own fields. The accommodation of men and women under the same roofs and the development of open relationships in highly liberal contexts have created much uproar in the region. Unlike in *Super Star*, participants in *Star Academy* lead their daily natural life under live camera and direct television transmission. Music coaching sessions are also transmitted live to allow viewers to contribute in the evaluation process. According to Kraidy (2005), *Star Academy* demonstrates that a television program can become a highly controversial public event that not only survives its numerous critics but at the same time saturates pan-Arab public discourse, becoming a full-fledged media event.

Million's Poet (Abu Dhabi Channel; year of launch: 2008). In this show, the best poet is chosen from a range of contestants who compete in what is described as the Arabs' biggest classical Arabic poetry reality show. Organized and produced by the Abu Dhabi Authority for Culture and Heritage, the show is broadcast live every Wednesday at 10:30 pm on Abu Dhabi TV. The competition between the poets normally gets tougher in the second phase as they are required to deliver a free rhyme poem from 15 verses in the first part of the episode. In the second part, contestants have to prove their poetical ability to build up a poem that keeps up with famous poems. In one episode, four female poets who participated in this season were able to make it to the second phase as they delivered powerful poems that impressed the jury panel and the audience. The *Million's Poet* who wins first place receives an increased grand prize of five million AED ($1,362,000) while the one ranking second receives four million AED ($1,090,000).

Stars of Science (Qatar Television; year of launch: 2009). In this show, 16 young Arab men and women from different backgrounds and professional/academic disciplines are selected by a professional jury of engineering, design, and business experts to take their innovation projects forward. Each contestant has an original project he/she wishes to turn into an innovation with real-life application. The 16 selected innovators work on their projects in a specially-designed workshop based inside Doha's innovation hub, Qatar Science and Technology Park, that is equipped with state-of-the-art tools, materials, and computer labs. During the weeks, contestants are tutored by experts in the business, and are given unprecedented levels of access to the resources and expertise from some of the world's finest academic institutions (Qatar Foundation, 2010).

Findings

Based on their moral worldviews, the 80 students who were randomly selected from 1200 College of Communication students to rate the presence of 10 values in the four "globalized" and "localized" reality shows they had watched. As Table 1 suggests, while students perceived some of the values to be generally shared by the two program categories, there were clear divergences about others. It is clear from the table that respondents reported the dominance of shared values like freedom, individualism, innovation, diversity, participation, and cooperation while they diverged on values like responsibility, decency, intimacy, and honor. While the first set of converging values may be labeled as universal proto-norms, diverging values are intrinsically culture-specific and are defined by the peculiar cultural and social context in which respondents live.

Table 1 summarizes students' views of both sets of programs.

TABLE 1
Students' views of both sets of programs (mean scores out of 5)

Value	Star Academy	Super Star	Million's Poet	Stars of Science
Freedom	4.2	4.1	4.0	3.8
Responsibility	2.0	1.5	4.2	4.5
Decency	1.4	2.1	3.9	3.8
Intimacy	4.2	3.8	2.1	1.8
Individualism	3.7	3.8	4.2	3.6
Innovation	3.6	3.5	4.3	4.6
Diversity	3.2	3.1	3.1	3.4
Honor	1.4	2.4	4.3	3.4
Participation	3.9	4.0	3.8	4.2
Cooperation	3.6	3.8	3.3	4.5

Freedom

Students perceived both "localized" and "globalized" television shows to carry a significant degree of freedom. Yet, based on the post-survey focus-group discussion, students were able to differentiate between two types of freedom in the four shows: in the globalized programs, it was freedom from the social and cultural shackles imposed on personal lifestyle. That was particularly conspicuous when it comes to men in close contact with women, putting on what students believe were indecent clothes, and even in practicing the very art of singing and music. On the other hand, a majority of students also saw the value of freedom in the localized programs in a different way. In both *Stars of Science* and the *Million's Poet*, it is freedom to be creative and to pursue your cultural visions through oral expression and scientific innovation. The basic impression I received from my post-survey focus-group discussion is that while "globalized" reality shows do promote freedom in its Western liberal sense, this type of freedom is not relevant to Arab communities, especially in the conservative Gulf region.

Responsibility

Based on their perceptions, students seemed unanimous in seeing "globalized" shows as least responsible when it comes to their representation of what they see as "cherished" social values and traditions. In the focus-group discussion following the survey, it was clear that most of the students viewed such shows as engaging in what some labeled "subversive" activities that seek to destroy our morality and force alien values and norms from outside. On the other hand, it was clear that the two "localized" shows were favorably viewed as highly responsible because, as students noted, the shows sought to revive our oral traditions and past scientific heritage through poetry and innovation. According to students taking part in the focus-group discussions, participants appearing in the two "localized" shows were demonstrating their commitment to the development of their nations and communities through indulgence in oral and scientific feats that are far more important than music and singing. Again, these perceptions of performing arts as constituting lower priorities when it comes to community development reflects a highly traditional view of what music can do in promoting social and cultural advancement in the Middle East.

Decency

Decency here refers to the quality of conforming to Arab-Islamic standards of propriety and morality. The view of both *Super Star* and *Star Academy* as carrying indecent features represented by participants' clothes and verbal and non-verbal language shows a rather conservative view of the public sphere. For some respondents taking part in the focus-group discussion, indecency also derives from the fact that young men and women are working very closely together with no barriers in the context of the performing arts. It was noted that the fact that women appearing in the "globalized" programs were wearing tight clothes with no head covers and with parts of their bodies exposed was bound to reflect a negative image of the two shows. On the other hand, mean scores for respondents' views of the two localized shows suggest how their conservative dress code and physical disengagement of men and women in public space were perceived as highly positive. One of the poets who appeared in the *Million's Poet* show was a Saudi woman (Hissa Hilal) who wore a veil and was introduced to the stage by a female presenter. In *Stars of Science*, there was only one young woman with no head cover and innovators were mingling in a "scientific exploration" rather than in a performing art context. This very context of the show seemed to have been quite central in defining students' perceptions of it as highly decent.

Intimacy

Describing close familiarity or association among participants in the shows, intimacy is one of the defining features of how ethical communication could be perceived in the Middle Eastern public sphere. It was clear that respondents perceived the two globalized formats showing significant intimate scenes or words relating to how men and women communicate. In one of the *Super Star* episodes, even the referee committee was so moved by the lyrics of one song because it was thought to be "too seductive" to overlook. In *Star Academy*, the fact that men and women are staying under the same roof under the camera spotlight was raising a lot of eyebrows among students. On the other hand, while some of the poems delivered on the *Million's Poet* carried highly sentimental elements, they were generally viewed as far more abstract than the visual messages embedded in the globalized programs. In the *Stars of Science*, intimacy received the lowest mean score because respondents perceived the show as purely scientific.

Individualism

Interestingly, the findings suggest that students perceived the two reality program categories as having a significant individualistic component. In the focus-group discussion, students were unanimous in describing each participant in the show, whether he/she is a performing artist, a poet, or a scientist, as seeking to reflect his/her individual self and to express his/her potential as a creative person in his/her field of specialty. Singers and actors on *Super Star* and *Star Academy* are after fame (and of course, fortune) and they see themselves as commanding a potential to realize their goals. In the *Million's Poet* and the *Stars of Science*, the notion of individualism is highly visible in the assertive and competitive feature of the program where each participant is harnessing his/own potential to beat his/her rivals. Of course, this does not mean that there is no place for collectivism in the shows. In fact, both *Stars of Science* and *Star Academy* participants do their work in a team-based style.

Innovation

Respondents reported the value of innovation embedded in the four reality television shows examined in this study. It is interesting to find that while the majority of respondents thought the globalized shows had negative effects on their communities by virtue of their promotion of Westernized lifestyles and values, they still believe it takes a good deal of creativity and innovation to produce competitive performing arts. This variation in perceptions of communication as "socially unacceptable" and as "creatively distinctive" is a significant finding that marks key tensions between the social and the innovative as not too mutually exclusive ingredients of communication acts. In the localized shows, students taking part in the focus-group discussion noted how poetry represents a talent that takes some creative power to induce in the dominantly oral Arab traditions. For the *Stars of Science* show, it was clear for respondents that the power to innovate was indispensible for giving rise to technological inventions. In many ways, the relationship between innovation, on the one hand, and poetic composition and scientific inventions, on the other hand, seems more acceptable than its relationship with performing arts, on the other hand, something that strikes at the very power of cultural peculiarity to define critical values and attitudes.

Diversity

Diversity here does not only denote a state of difference, but recognition of that difference as healthy. Respondents' views of diversity in the four shows were generally rated as "high". The "globalized" shows hosted young men and women from different ages and nationalities and their performances reflected such pluralistic composition. It should be noted that for viewers of the globalized reality programs, the issue was often turning into one of patriotism as they voted for their favorite stars. Hence, the two programs were turning into arenas for national competition among stars affiliated with nationally and geographically divergent publics. For the *Million's Poet* respondents perceived diversity to be manifested in the wide-ranging topics addressed by poets, their national affiliation, and their gender composition. The final decisions on winners rested with a referee committee made up of poetry critics. The same criteria seemed to have been applied to the *Stars of Science* show where participants hailed from different Arab countries, pursued different scientific feats, and were marked by good gender composition.

Honor

Honor is one of the central cultural values defining Arabs' worldview (Ayish and Badawi, 1997). In many ways, honor is associated with a good public reputation that derives from decency in the person's conduct and of his relatives, especially women. It is in this context that respondents thought the globalized shows which feature women with clothing which left parts of their bodies exposed as low in honor. They thought that no matter how noble the theme of the performing arts is, it should be delivered in the most decent and honorable forms. In the poetry and science programs, respondents believed it was "honorable" to compose poetry and defend one's reputation and that of his tribal or national leaders. It was also "honorable" to pursue scientific and technological innovations because that would eventually enhance the development of their communities. This view of poetry and scientific invention as "honorable" acts that deserve to be supported is reinforced by the fact that both shows are delivered in a context with high cultural and social relevance.

Participation

For many respondents, the fact that average persons with outstanding talents are enabled to express their creative powers in performing arts, poetry and scientific innovations is a positive development in a region long marked by state-controlled access to the public sphere. This view has been noted in writings by Ayish (2009) and Kraidy (2007) about reality television promoting democratic participation in the Arab world. In perceptions of the four shows, it was clear that the new Arab public sphere carries a good promise for non-mainstream voices to be heard on the basis of their personal creative merits rather than on the basis of their political or ethnic features. In the focus-group discussion, students seemed unanimous in noting how reality shows are empowering talented persons to find their way into achievement, something that is barely present in real-world situations in the region. This sense of participatory orientation, according to students, would most likely contribute to the diffusion of a new democratic culture in which the individual makes the aspired difference.

Cooperation

In the Middle East's consensus-based political and cultural traditions, conflict is viewed as a negative quality that would most likely hinder community progress. The extent to which the four reality shows demonstrate cooperation as a defining value has received almost similar ratings by students, at least in the *Star Academy*, *Super Star* and the *Million's Poet* shows. But it also generated higher ratings in the *Stars of Science* show because all scientific inventions are achievable only through team work. In the focus-group discussion, students noted that even performing arts are team-based feats that need to be carried out on the basis of concerted efforts exerted by musicians, performers, and even the studio-based audience. The same applies to the poetry program which is intrinsically centered on the poet himself; yet, the role of the referee panel and the audience is also instrumental in defining the final outcome of the competition. In the *Stars of Science* show, it was impossible for one young scientist to come up with any invention on his or her own. The division of labor within teams required contributions from all members to realize the final innovation and explain it before the panel of judges.

Conclusion

The findings of this study suggest that Arab publics' perceptions of "globalized" and "localized" reality television shows do not carry clear-cut demarcations between what is ethically good or bad. The fact that students believe the two program categories share six values and diverge on four others is quite significant for addressing global media ethics in the region. As noted earlier, the converging values in students' responses actually represent universal proto-norms that are shared across cultures while the diverging values are intrinsically cultural and suggest some peculiarity to the region's religious and social traditions. The fact that students saw "globalized" and "localized" reality shows as carrying both global and local values is important for the glocalization or hybridization of media ethics. This study demonstrates that it is difficult to think of media ethics beyond their local and global dimensions but as harmoniously integrated into a new system of "glocalized" media ethics. The study concludes that public perceptions of media ethics are rooted in local and global grounds and this should serve as a catalyst for media professionals to understand universals in undertaking future ethical initiatives.

REFERENCES

AL JAZEERA (2008) "Code of Ethics", http://english.aljazeera.net/aboutus/2006/11/20085251857 33692771.html, accessed 10 June 2010.

AL KAAKI, AZZA (2008) "Reality Television Shows Effects on the Young in Qatar", paper presented to the conference on communication and globalization, Sultan Qaboos University, Muscat, 21–23 November.

AMIN, HUSSEIN (2008) "The Arab States Charter for Satellite Television: a quest for regulation", *Arab Media & Society*, March, http://www.arabmediasociety.com/?article =649, accessed 15 May 2010.

ARAB ADVISORS GROUP (2008) *Arab Reality TV Shows: a strategic report* I, Amman, Jordan: Arab Advisors Group.

ARAB ADVISORS GROUP (2010) *Arab Reality TV Shows: a strategic report* II, Amman, Jordan: Arab Advisors Group.

AYISH, MUHAMMAD (2008) "Reality Television and Its Effects and Youth and the Family in the GCC region", paper presented to the conference on satellite television and the moral challenge, Doha, Qatar, 2–3 November.

AYISH, MUHAMMAD (2009) "Reality TV Is Good for Arab Democracy", *Daily Star (Beirut)*, 16 March, p. 11.

AYISH, MUHAMMAD and BADAWI, HAYDAR (1997) "The Arab-Islamic Heritage in Communication Ethics", in: Cliff Christians and Michael Traber (Eds), *Communication Ethics and Universal Values*, Thousand Oaks, CA: Sage, pp. 105–27.

CHRISTIANS, CLIFF, RAO, SHAKUNTALA, WARD, STEPHEN and WASSERMAN, HERMAN (2008) "Toward a Global Media Ethics: theoretical perspectives", *Ecquid Novi: African Journalism Studies* 29(2), pp. 135–72.

CHRISTIANS, CLIFF and TRABER, MICHAEL (Eds) (1997) *Communication Ethics and Universal Values*, Thousand Oaks, CA: Sage.

DOHA DECLARATION (2008) "Declaration on the Effects of Satellite Television on Youth in the GCC Region", Doha, Qatar, 2–3 November.

INTERNATIONAL FEDERATION OF JOURNALISTS (IFJ) (2010) "The Ethical Journalism Initiative", http:// ethicaljournalisminitiative.org/en, accessed 21 December 2010.

KRAIDY, MARWAN (2005) "Reality Television and Politics in the Arab World: preliminary observations", *Transnational Broadcasting Journal*(online), Fall, http://www.tbsjournal. com/Archives/Fall05/Kraidy.html, accessed 15 February 2010.

KRAIDY, MARWAN (2007) "Reality Television and Democratization in the Arab World", in: Isaac Blankson and Patrick Murphy (Eds), *Negotiating Democracy: media transformations in emerging democracies*, New York: State University of New York Press, pp. 179–98.

KRAIDY, MARWAN (2009) *Reality Television and Arab Politics: contentions in public life*, Cambridge: Cambridge University Press.

QATAR FOUNDATION (2010) "Stars of Science", http://starsofscience.com/sos/en/program_concept. asp, accessed 20 January 2011.

RAO, SHAKUNTALA and WASSERMAN, HERMAN (2007) "Postcolonial Theory and Global Media Ethics: a theoretical intervention", paper presented to the International Roundtable on Global Media Ethics, Stellenbosch, South Africa.

ROBERTSON, RONALD (1995) "Glocalization: time-space and homogeneity heterogeneity", in: Mike Featherstone, Scott Lash and Ronald Robertson (Ed.), *Global Modernities*, London: Sage, pp. 25–44.

STEINER, LINDA (2011) "The Value of (Universal) Values in the Work of Clifford Christians", *Journal of Mass Media Ethics* 25(2), pp. 110–20.

TEHRANIAN, MAJID (2002) "Peace Journalism", *The Harvard International Journal of Press/Politics* 9(2), pp. 58–83.

WARD, STEPHEN (2005) "Philosophical Foundations for a Global Journalism Ethics", *Journal of Mass Media Ethics* 20(1), pp. 3–21.

WARD, STEPHEN (2008) "Global Journalism Ethics: widening the conceptual base", *Global Media Journal (Canadian Edition)* 1(1), pp. 137–49.

WASSERMAN, HERMAN and RAO, SHAKUNTALA (2008) "The Glocalization of Journalism Ethics", *Journalism* 9(2), pp. 163–81.

THE "LOCAL" IN GLOBAL MEDIA ETHICS

Shakuntala Rao

This article explores critical regionalism, as defined in the works of Gayatri Chakravorty Spivak, as a way to understand and expand the concept of "local" in global media ethics. By using examples of South Asian media, the essay concludes that the epistemic inclusion of critical regionalism, contextualized within the broader disciplinary position of Postcolonial theory, can enrich our understanding of the nexus of media ethics, localization, and identity politics.

Introduction

In the past two decades, liberalization and privatization of the media systems, first in Europe and North America and then in the countries of the South, has created a new media world order. The existing centers of power for the past few centuries—be it the European nations of Britain, France, Spain, and Italy and the post-World War II United States—are currently renegotiating their place in world history and in increasingly transnational media flows. The old categories which had defined international communication are passé. The rise of "Chindia" (the joint economic and political powerhouses of China and India); the post-apartheid rise of South Africa; Middle East nations', such as United Arab Emirates, Qatar, Bahrain, and Saudi Arabia, with their vast repositories of natural resources; and the post-Soviet Russia's resurgent military and cultural dominance over Eastern Europe and Asian Republics challenge and render obsolete previous descriptions of the global media landscape. The focus of academic work in communication, media studies, and journalism has shifted from a paradigm of international communication to one of media globalization where cultural, economic, political, social, and technical analysis of communication patterns and effects between nations has given way to studies of exchanges between transnational corporations, local and regional media companies, consumers, and media workers (Thussu, 2006).

Given contemporary globalization, I argue that the course of global media ethics must move towards an epistemic reorientation of studying media narratives' production, reception, and consumption. Using the recent works of postcolonial theorist, Gayatri Chakravorty Spivak, I advocate for "critical regionalism" (2008, p. 99) to map a new understanding of the "local" in global media ethics. Though the burgeoning literature on global media ethics has begun to question the conflation of local and regional with national, the concept of "local" by and large remains ill-defined (Rao and Wasserman, 2007). Much of the writing in global media ethics has concerned itself with universals and proto-norms and the discussions about the local has sometimes been relegated to philosophical and cultural relativism. While universals need to be centralized by media ethicists as new technologies converge, the "local" cannot be lost or reductively analyzed, in the sharp rhetoric of anti-relativism. One must resist, as Christians et al. (2008, p. 159) write, "the relentless and irresistible tendency of universalization that has plagued global media ethics." At the heart is the "inequality of global traffic of knowledge production and distribution" (Shome, 2009, p. 695) which valorizes some local knowledge as universals and imprisons other knowledge as relative. Using South Asian media as an example, I argue for the epistemic inclusion of critical regionalism as a way to extend and enrich our understanding of the nexus of global media ethics, localization, and identity politics.

Communication, Media Studies and Postcolonial Theory

In communication and media studies, debates have been raging about the complex and contradictory influences of the global media industries on local identities, cultures, and ideologies. Recent trends toward concentration of media ownership deregulation and new alliances between transnational media corporations and national governments are changing the nature of media content and practices (Hafez, 2007). Journals and monographs in communication, media and journalism studies have been inundated with theories attempting to explain the dramatic changes in the global media scene. One theory consistently advocated has been a kind of "bureaucratic rationalization or McDonaldization" (Sparks, 2000, p. 78), an analysis in which the takeover of locally-owned media and other similar inflow of foreign capital has been seen as "the progressive erosion of local media and their incorporation into, or replacement by, larger predators" (Sparks, 2000, p. 78). While the study of global media has historically emphasized media and cultural imperialism—especially inaugurated in the works of Schiller and Hamelink—these explanations emphasized a one-way media flow. Hamelink, in the introduction of his book *Cultural Autonomy in Global Communication*, wrote "The process of cultural synchronization implies that a particular type of cultural development in the metropolitan country is persuasively communicated to the receiving country. The metropolis offers the model with which the receiving parties synchronize" (1983, p. 5). While the scholarly gaze was on whatever the presumptively imperialistic foreign content does to the local people, the local people were characterized as passive victims rather than as agents of their local appropriations of the foreign, however complicitous with or resistant to hegemonic ideologies. There had been a failure to recognize the fraught, tense, uneven, and shifting reciprocity between the global and the local.

Scholars such as Appadurai and others have begun to critique such assumptions. In his essay titled "Disjuncture and Difference in the Global Culture Economy", Appadurai (1994) centralizes and problematizes the inherent tension between homogenization and heterogenization. He argues that global cultural process is fundamentally characterized by "radical disjunctures between different sorts of global flows and the uncertain landscapes created in and through these disjuncture" (Appadurai, 1994, p. 296). "Modernity as rupture" is constituted by, for Appadurai (1994, p. 297), the joint work of media and migration. The global movement of media technologies into every aspect of individual lives and the unprecedented mass migration of peoples across the world together define "the core of the link between globalization and the modern" (Appadurai, 1994, p. 297). Media and migration, both separately and together, produce an enormous degree of instability in the creation of selves and identities.

I find that Postcolonial theory offers concepts that can help us think about this dynamic relation between the global and the local in communication and media studies. Shome and Hegde's (2002) essay titled, "Postcolonial Approaches to Communication:

charting the terrain, engaging the intersections", in the special issue of *Communication Theory*, speaks of merging the rich literature in Postcolonial theory to communication as a way to provide some epistemological questions and answers. Communication and media scholars, Shome and Hegde observe, have continued to valorize views of media and culture rooted in the West which have remained predominantly influenced by modernist intellectual and institutional structures. For Shome and Hegde, it is the epistemic reorientation of media studies which is necessary in order to enter any cogent discussions of the global/local dialectic. Their starting point is the fast changing and overly mediated social and cultural formations dominating our world and linking these changes to history, power, space, and politics. If one is to proceed with academic responsibility, they argue, communication scholars must include representation, identity, hybridity, and agency in their discussions and analyses. By invoking the critical vein of Postcolonial theory, these authors urge the readers to take communication and media studies out of the parochialism of theory steeped in Eurocentrism that "either ignores completely or oversimplifies the complexity of the rest" (Shome and Hegde, 2002, p. 260). Postcolonial theorists, Shome and Hegde write, understand the current global order is not "born fully-formed, Minerva style" but comes to us situated within the larger historical sweep of colonialism and its imperial centers (2002, p. 261). I do not assume that Postcolonial theory (as opposed to Feminism, Marxism, or Poststructuralism) provides the only resources to scholars in global media ethics, but the concept of critical regionalism strikes me as particularly useful.

The emergence of colonial and postcolonial studies within the academy as a distinct mode of critical analysis can be dated to the end of the 1970s, perhaps best periodized with the publication of Said's book *Orientalism* (1978). The concurrent works of Bhabha on hybridity, mimcry, and mimesis and Spivak's essays on subaltern politics, situated in the disciplines of English and comparative literature, asked provocative questions about representation, language, power, and knowledge, and abstractly engaged the problem of ways to begin to grasp the relationship between the colonial/imperial and nationalist past and the circumstances and the exigencies of the present. As Young (2001, p. 88) has pointed out, postcolonialism examines "the material and epistemological conditions of postcoloniality and seeks to combat the continuing, often covert, operation of an imperialist system of economic, political, and cultural domination." Postcolonialism should not be taken as an "endorsement of the new world system"; it is a "radical response to its condition" (Ashcroft, 2001, p. 24). While the label "postcolonialism", like any term that ends in "ism" describing a critical enterprise, implies a homogeneous ideology, theoretical perspective, and political agenda, its name contradicts its divergent actual critical practices. All critical practices that go under the name of postcolonialism, however, have sought to dismantle the West as the normative center of the world, to move beyond West-centered historicism, beyond imperial binary structures of Self/Other and center/periphery, and ultimately beyond any form of imperialism. Such theory can help us create an epistemology for media and journalism studies that also deconstructs hegemonic Western notions about a globalized media.

It is only recently that theorists have attempted to engage postcolonial studies in contemporary global terms. Globalization does not exist outside history, "in a kind of universal postmodern space" (Spivak, 2003, p. 80); globalization also reveals itself best as the site of practices and strategies which have been developed by local communities over many centuries. We cannot understand globalization without understanding the structure of global power relations which flourishes in the twenty-first century as an economic, cultural, and political legacy of Western imperialism (ideas which are at the core of the postcolonial disciplinary stance). Postcolonial theory can provide clear models for understanding how local communities achieve agency under the pressures of global hegemony. Postcolonial theorists resist the common view, often purported by the academic left, that "globalization is simply re-colonization" (Xie, 2006, p. 71). To the contrary, the engagement of local communities with global culture is marked by a great degree of self-determination and creative interpolation of local empowerment in the face of dominant hegemonic discourse. Postcolonial theory offers intellectual critique and countervailing ethics for the new eco-environmental issues, electronic media and networks, and increased mobility of peoples. Spivak and others have tried to shift the debates in Postcolonial theory from the study of "metropolitan multicultural phenomenon" (Spivak, 2008, p. 101) to more regional and local issues, often situated outside of Western academies and institutions.

In recent times, communication, media and journalism studies have been inundated with questions about the "ethical" and the enduring nature of certain philosophical problems. There has even been a "turn to ethics" in a number of disciplines (Garber et al., 2000, p. viii); this raises the question of what one turns from in order to arrive at the ethical. The inevitable answer to this question would be a turn away from the political. If the turn to ethics is a turn away from political, Postcolonial theory can help ground us back in the professional practice of media, the philosophical questions such practices raise, understand the historical location of mediated relations, and the immediacy of their effects. Studies in global media ethics must then be understood, not merely as "fantasy" but truly transformative in the way media professionals practice and impact on the social world. This is often difficult. Outside the academy it is very arduous for media professionals and journalists, primarily because of time and resource constraints, to engage in lengthy and vigilant interpretations of philosophical questions and study research developed over many decades. Quite often one hears journalists say that scholars studying media ethics are too busy imposing upon them a joyless vigilance (clothed in a language of intellectual expertise) rather than providing constructive analyses of professional practices and outcomes. The scope of global media ethics can be a turn to the ethical in a way that bridges such polarity; it can also provide a basis of political action which is ethical in its very enterprise.

Critical Regionalism: The "Local" in Communication, Journalism, and Media Studies

One of the defining features of the twenty-first century is the increasingly convoluted and complex interplay between localism and globalism, and its implications for disciplinary boundaries. Clearly, this process has been in operation for centuries, but its velocity has risen sharply during the past 50 years. The interaction has produced remarkable transformations in the spaces of politics, economics, and culture, as newer forms of capital began to imprint their local visibilities and inflect on locality (and nation) in unanticipated ways. A productive way to understand the dialectic between the global and the local, writes Dissanayake (2006, p. 26), is through "an examination of the production of newer and more complex localities." Whenever scholars seek to interrogate the intersecting narratives of the global and the local, what they are hoping to do is to focus on the production of the local and its ever-changing contours in response to the imperatives of the global. The local is never static; its boundaries, both temporal and spatial, are subject to ceaseless change. The local is characterized by a web of power plays, agonistic interest, pluralized histories, and the struggle over polysemic and asymmetrical exchanges. The local is constantly transforming and reinventing itself as it seeks to reach beyond itself and engage the translocal. The question, "What is local?" has remained at the center of disciplinary conversations as theorists struggle with notions of justice, tolerance, and coexistence. Spivak (2008, p. 95), in the essay "1994: will postcolonialism travel?", tackles the most challenging question of our times: "What kind of a collective are we part of or on what plain can we be imagined as a collectivity?" She carefully charts the idea of critical regionalism which I want to elucidate for our use in global media ethics.

Various new spatial keywords—regionalism, regionalization, territorial complexes, deterritorialized publics, borderlands, glocalisms, transregional—have come to the fore in humanities and social sciences because they seem especially well suited to an analysis of present-day restructurings. In one of the first usages of critical regionalism, geographer Soja saw its analytic power to bear upon the reconceptualization of the local and then working through it to formulate theories of "newer global communities and relations" (1989, p. 31). Regionalism as a scholarly area of interest has itself been a remarkably diffuse concept. A term that has currency, but different values in political science, urban planning, architecture and design, history, literature, and visual arts. More recently, regionalism has moved beyond being perceived merely as a geophysical entity to an emerging scholarship which shifts the emphasis away from the products of regional culture to the processes by which ideas about regions come into being and become influential. Instead of asking whether a particular version of region is valid or invalid, authentic or not, "critical regionalism asks whose interests are served by a given version of the region" (Powell, 2007, p. 22).

Spivak borrows the term from Frampton (2002, p. 78), whose academic work in architecture forms the basis for its use in other disciplines. As an architect, Frampton was appalled by what he viewed as the increasing "megalopolitan development" of large cities lined with free-standing high-rises and serpentine highways. Architecture, Frampton wrote, can only be sustained today as a critical practice if it assumes an "arriere-garde position", one which distances itself equally from the Enlightenment myth of progress and from a reactionary unrealistic impulse to "return to the architonic forms of the pre-industrial past" (2002, p. 81). The fundamental strategy of critical regionalism in architecture, for Frampton, mediates the impact of universal civilization with elements derived directly from the peculiarities of a particular place. "The practice of critical regionalism is contingent upon a process of double mediation," writes Frampton, "it has to 'deconstruct' the overall spectrum of world culture which it inevitably inherits and it has to achieve, through synthetic contradiction, a manifest critique of universal civilization" (2002, p. 83). For critical regionalism in architecture, local topography and nature was integrated into the structures one builds; the site—signs of its history in geological, archeological, and agricultural terms—becomes inscribed in the design and realization of the built structure. Critical regionalism in architecture acknowledges, and tries to alleviate, what Heidegger (1975, p. 154) called the "loss of nearness" characteristic of built structures of global modernity.

Spivak's use of the architectural strategy of critical regionalism is partly based on Heidegger's plea of renewing "nearness." Critical regionalism, in Spivak's work, is connected to the view that Asia (as a Continent) needs to be pluralized; that Asia singular must become conceptualized as "other Asias", as the title of her book suggests. Spivak observes that we know little about "areas that are not immediately in our experience, areas that general official histories have marginalized" (2008, p. 95). While she was growing up in post-independence India of the 1950s, she knew more about European and American culture and politics than about those of adjoining Asian nations. Although they did not play out in geopolitical realms and among policy mavens, the historically strong regional connections, Spivak (2008, p. 95) writes, "lingered in cultural memory." In *Other Asias*, Spivak focuses on a question posed by two scholars, Kassabian and Kazanjian, "Why is there no Armenian postcolonialism?" (2008, p. 99). Here Spivak acknowledges the limits of postcolonialism thus far. Focusing on Armenia requires a renewed understanding of Said's Orientalism and postcolonialism; she says, "It is a different kind of postcoloniality that we have in those areas. It is not a repetition of the Victorian model of the division between public and private" (Spivak, 2008, p. 275). Given that the Southern caucuses and Central Asia are looking at the displacement of the Soviet Union into the Russian Federation, postcolonial questions do not fit neatly on to Armenia. Spivak writes:

> Armenia cannot lean towards existing theories. It cannot be comfortably located in the generally recognized lineaments of contemporary imperialism and received postcoloni-alism. Its history is diversified, with many loyalties crosshatching so small a place. (2008, p. 117)

To locate Armenia within the larger grid of crisscrossing identities and histories is to practice "othering ourselves into many Asias" and to release Asia, and Asian thinkers, from hermetically sealed identities of being "Asians" but locate Asia as a contested site of multiple hierarchies, genealogies, national, and ethnic histories superimposed by colonialism, genocide (her example here is the centrality of Armenian genocide of 1915), and modernity (2008, p. 211). The only way out, Spivak argues, is to advocate for an anti-ethnic regionalism that displaces ethnic histories but reterritorializes regional histories and also moves us "a step beyond the nation-state" (2008, p. 233). Critical regionalism is not about a space or site—which makes her use of the concept different from that of Frampton—but naming of a "critical position" (2008, p. 235) through a pedagogy of "genealogical deconstruction" which makes it possible for other Asias, other Africas, and other globes to erase the "regionalist unilateralism of Euro-US and diasporic hegemony" (2008, p. 238). The route to "rewriting postcolonialism into globality through critical regionalism" needs a rigorous intellectual path focused on epistemic and ethical pluralization, not simply recognition of cultural difference (Spivak, 2008, p. 131). When we talk about a region, in critical regionalism, we are not talking about a stable, boundaried, autonomous place but about a cultural history, the cumulative, generative effect of the interplay among the various, competing definitions of that region. Critical regionalism understood in this sense places importance on the grassroots, of a vigorous generative understanding of the local, of social action and movements, in short, critical regionalism can be the construction of region to interconnect more fully, rather than disconnect, local places to broader patterns of politics, history, and culture.

Critical Regionalism, South Asia, and Media Ethics

As we acknowledge the positionality of other Asias, we must reconfigure if the "local" in communication, media and journalism studies must go over and beyond the nation into new forms of collectivities. For instance, studying Bollywood films (Hindi films made in Mumbai in India) requires understanding of varied and highly diverse transnational audiences; the "local" in Bollywood audience studies includes audiences all over the world. Kaur and Sinha's (2005, p. 1) descriptive term of "Bollyworld" challenges the utter absurdity in trying to fix audiences to a singular locale (Hindi-speaking audiences in India), as these films routinely play to sold out crowds in Dakar, Dubai, Cairo, Johannesburg, and Toronto. While critical regionalism supplements the notion of "cultural proximity" (Straubhaar, 2007, p. 23) in media consumption and production, it also assumes a fundamental of the postcolonial stance: the shared meaning of historical experiences and imaginations. The "local" must then get reterritorialized and historicized outside of lineaments of nation and ethnic nationalism to a different kind of collective. I chose to use media in South Asia in this analysis because it can provide us with frames of intelligibilities, repertoire of images, and enfolding discourses that can enable us to make greater sense of the interanimation of the global and the local. While using South Asia as a starting point, I believe the analysis can be easily extended to other contested regions such as the Middle East, Africa, and Russia.

I begin with a question: What is South Asia? A Wikipedia list includes the nations of India, Bangladesh, Pakistan, Bhutan, Sri Lanka, and Nepal. What the Wikipedia list does not include are the sub-states—with quotation marks around them—of Tamil Eelam, Kashmir, and North West frontier province in Pakistan. Defining South Asia—as in Spivak's chagrin in defining Asia diversified—requires the conscious marginalization of nation as providing linear and policed cultural parameters. The new vocabulary of critical regionalism requires reconfiguring the kind of collectives which have existed and might evolve in South Asia.

Sub-national regionalism has been an integral part of a historic pre-colonial identity in South Asia. For instance, the partition of the Indian subcontinent in 1947 led to the divisions of the Punjab province into two new provinces: East and West Punjab. The predominantly Sikh and Hindu East Punjab became part of the new nation of India while the predominantly Muslim West Punjab became part of Pakistan. Punjabis in both nations continued to share the same language, Punjabi, and have close cultural affiliations. Similarly, Bengal, a historical and geographical region in northeast South Asia, was divided into West and East Bengal. Today East Bengal is the independent nation of Bangladesh and the state of West Bengal is part of India. The majority of West Bengal and Bangladesh is inhabited by people who speak Bengali and make up the ethno-linguistic region of Bengal. In Sri Lanka, the minority population of Tamilians share their ethno-linguistic heritage with people from the Southern state of Tamil Nadu in India. The Liberation Tigers of Tamil Eelam referred to as LTTE (or Tamil Tigers) has been a militant organization that has waged a violent secessionist campaign against the Sri Lankan government (dominated by the Buddhist Sinhalese Sri Lankans) since the early 1970s to create their own Tamil state. The most powerful political party in Tamil Nadu, the DMK (Dravida Munnetra Kazhagam), has had strong LTTE leanings. Such examples testify that the idea of region is in many ways categorically different from other conceptualizations of place, like home, community, city, State, and nation, in that region does not refer to a specific site but to a larger network of sites; region is always a relational term; at any site on the landscape, multiple definitions of place are continually in play and at work, sometimes convivially and sometimes antagonistically.

A visit to a town like Janakpur, like a close look at the complicated history of Armenia, alerts us both to the problematics of cultural, political, and linguistic boundaries of the postcolonial state and possibilities for critical regionalism. About 10 miles from the Indian border, Janakpur is the capital of the region of Terai, part of the southeastern plains of Nepal, and a Hindu holy city signified by the massive presence of the Janaki Temple in the city square. The area has close connections with the northeastern Indian state of Bihar which borders Terai, but the town, with a population of less than 100,000, is far away from the geopolitical "nations" of Nepal and India. People in Nepal who speak Maithili and Bhojpuri and call themselves the Madeshis live primarily in Terai. Maithili and Bhojpuri are also the two dominant languages of Bihar. Like Biharis, Madeshis are predominantly Hindus, as opposed to the Newars of Katmandu Valley who are Buddhists, with a belief that Sita, the consort of Rama from the Indian epic of Ramayana, was a Maithili princess from the region.

A long-standing socio-political movement in the Terai region, under different names and political leaderships, has been fighting for rights and recognition for the Madeshis since the 1950s. Until recently the movement had been defined by Nepal's monarchy (and, subsequently, by the democratic governments) as an ethno-linguistic movement; but movement leaders were actually primarily focused on land and cultural rights of the population. While the movement had had some violent factions, such as the Janatantrik Terai Mukti Morcha under the leadership of Jai Krishna Goit aligned to the Maoist guerillas who were waging an armed struggle against the Nepali monarchy, the Madeshi movement has largely been a peaceful one based on land rights. Says Uday Yadav, one of the leaders of the movement:

> Colonization of Madesh and Madeshi identity became essential [for Nepalis]. Exclusionary nationalism became the foundation of the modern Nepali state. Before the advent of democracy, the design of Shahas and Ranas for a Nepali state have been feudalistic in nature. The political elites after 1990 have further built on that. While the seizure of state power from the King provided the base for a new nationalism, the colonization of Madesh provides the economic base for reinforcing rule of the country by the Nepalis. From the very beginning, Madesh has been placed at the service of Nepalis. (personal communication, January 2008)

In the past few years Girija Prasad Koirala, first Prime Minister of post-monarchial democratic Nepal, had pursued radical land reform programs along the principles of democratic socialism in the Terai region. He intended to institutionalize the peasant economy in Terai and in Nepal. According to Yadav, however, Koirala refused to share the same egalitarian approach of land reform to political representation of the Madeshi. Most of the land seized by the state has either been given to Nepali hill migrants known as sukumbasi or continues to be under state control. Madeshi landless people remained dispossessed under new land reform policies of the state. In fact, the new citizenship act pending in the Nepal parliament might de-recognize some Madeshis. Madeshis, in organizing their social movements, have long taken cues from similar land rights movements in Bihar in India where the landless continue to face profound oppression, as do the Madeshis in Nepal. While these communities are connected ethnically and linguistically, they are also connected historically by their marginalization (both Terai and Bihar have been marginalized in state policies of Nepal and India, respectively) and in seeking demands for political representation, cultural autonomy, and land rights. Yadav acknowledges the influence of Bihari social movements such as those launched by the Ekta Parishad, an organization committed to the philosophy of Mahatma Gandhi of redistribution of lands to the landless and Bhoomi Sena, a group formed by the lower castes of Bihari Kumris, on Madeshi movements.

To reconfigure the local in South Asian media and to adopt the epistemic project of critical regionalism, scholars must focus on places like Janakpur. In Janakpur, houses along the narrow streets of the bazaar leading from the Janaki Temple are littered with satellite dishes receiving a number channels from Nepal and India with the most popular being the general news and entertainment channel in Bhojpuri called Mahuaa TV. The one movie theater in Janakpur plays Bhojpuri films produced in Patna, the capital city of Bihar. Janak FM, the local radio station, carries news programs, songs, and talk-shows in Maithili, Bhojpuri, Hindi, and Nepali. For media scholars, an overt focus on the structure of global media networks located in the Western hemisphere will not work in Janakpur. There is no CNN, BBC, or STAR TV here. Similarly, there is no presence of state-owned television and radio. Even Bollywood, the largest film industry in South Asia, with its own preoccupation of reimagining the national space, is absent. The one Maithali newspaper published from Janakpur, *Hamra Nepal* (Our Nepal), focuses on water and other environmental issues and the Maoist movement which has affected farming communities on both sides of the border. News on Janak FM is an hourly bulletin where journalists report from Kathmandu, Delhi, and Patna. As in many non-media centric societies, a person's experience with media in Janakpur may comprise a small percentage of his or her total experience facilitated more by other institutions such as religion, education, and government. I suggest that critical regionalism in journalism and media studies begins by de-anchoring the geopolitical location of such audiences, understands their historical links to other regional/ethnic communities, understands the postcolonial condition in which these communities live, govern themselves, and seek self-determination, and the role, if any, the media play in grassroots communication and activism and in forming cross-border alliances. The ethical project for media scholars would include giving voices and to reinvigorate neglected contacts that already exist, investing a socially and spatially constructed idea of region with agency and purpose, to open the intellectual project to local participation specifically instructed by the voices and experiences of those normally excluded from powerful strands of public discourse, and survey the range of representational strategies for defining places and regions expressed or implied in a variety of media artifacts. Continuing to equate the "local" with the nation suppresses a more complicated matrix of ethno-linguistic, regional, communal, provincial, caste, gender, class, education, spatial, and historical connections. These interstices of regional connections serve the powerful functions of establishing cultural memory and identity through multiple layers of media consumption and production.

Christians (2008) is right to point out that media ethics education has been overly focused on the professional practices of journalists rather than grounding them in larger questions of morality. Past scholarly work in global media ethics has rightly tried to extend itself beyond the narrow confines of national media and merely studies of codes of ethics or parochial professional practices. Such efforts, though laudable, must not take us too far from the "local" and from ethical practices that define local action and politics. Central to the advocacy of the concept of critical regionalism, and its possible use in media ethics, is the epistemic and ontological need to undo a regime which had historically violated the alterity of the other, a regime that created false "national" boundaries and borders between peoples though such borders have never been able to annihilate the cultural history people continued to share. Critical regionalism and its disciplinary home of Postcolonial theory, posits that matters of subjectivity and identity must not only be addressed locally, relationally, and historically but that ethicists spend time in studying connections between peoples across borders.

In the advocacy of critical regionalism it is also necessary to isolate the question of otherness interpreted as multi-ethics, if indeed the elusive noun ethics bears being used in the plural. It is not an ethics about the other, but also ethics belonging to the other, or more precisely, others. From this position it follows that a radical democratic project of the region or local would involve not merely the cohabitation of multiple cultures, ethnic groups, or identities, with their respective claims to authenticity, equal dignity, respect, rights, or economic equity; the challenge relates also to how the coexistence of many versions of ethos, ethical habits, conventions, gestures, and substantivist narratives about the "good life" was still possible. Critical regionalism, and its use in global media ethics, must then move away from notions of balkanizations and culture wars with their bellicose intent and notions that media merely represent others, but to retrieve the alterity of the other in a pluralistic, non-violent, and emancipatory way.

REFERENCES

APPADURAI, ARJUN (1994) "Disjuncture and Difference in the Global Cultural Economy", in: Michael Featherstone (Ed.), *Global Culture: nationalism, globalization, and modernity*, London: Sage, pp. 295–310.

ASHCROFT, BILL (2001) *Post-colonial Transformation*, London: Routledge.

CHRISTIANS, CLIFFORD (2008) "Media Ethics in Education", *Journalism Communication Monographs* 9(4), pp. 181–221.

CHRISTIANS, CLIFFORD, RAO, SHAKUNTALA, WARD, STEPHEN and WASSERMAN, HERMAN (2008) "Toward a Global Media Ethics: theoretical perspectives", *Ecquid Novi: African Journalism Studies* 29(2), pp. 135–72.

DISSANAYAKE, WIMAL (2006) "Globalization and the Experience of Culture: the resilience of nationhood", in: Natascha Gentz and Stefan Kramer (Eds), *Globalization, Cultural Identities, and Media Representations*, Albany: State University of New York Press, pp. 25–44.

FRAMPTON, KENNETH (2002) *Labor, Work and Architecture: collected essays on architecture and design*, New York: Phaidon Press.

GARBER, MARJORIE, HANSSEN, BEATRICE and WALKOWITZ, REBECCA (2000) "Introduction: the turn to ethics", in: Marjorie Garber, Beatrice Hanssen and Rebecca Walkowitz (Eds), *The Turn to Ethics*, New York: Routledge, pp. vii–xii.

HAFEZ, KIA (2007) *The Myth of Media Globalization*, A. Skinner (Trans.), New York: Polity Press.

HAMELINK, CEES (1983) *Cultural Autonomy in Global Communication*, New York: Addison, Wesley, Longman.

HEIDEGGER, MARTIN (1975) *Poetry, Language, Thought*, New York: Harper Collins.

KAUR, RAMINDER and SINHA, AJAY (2005) "Bollyworld: an introduction to popular Indian cinema through a transnational lens", in: Raminder Kaur and Ajay Sinha (Eds), *Bollyworld: popular Indian cinema through a transnational lens*, New Delhi: Sage, pp. 1–12.

POWELL, DOUGLAS (2007). *Critical Regionalism: connecting politics and culture in the American landscape*, Chapel Hill: University of North Carolina Press.

RAO, SHAKUNTALA and WASSERMAN, HERMAN (2007) "Global Media Ethics Revisited: a postcolonial critique", *Journal of Global Media and Communication* 3(1), pp. 29–50.

SAID, EDWARD (1978) *Orientalism*, New York: Pantheon Books.

SHOME, RAKA (2009) "Post-colonial Reflections on the 'Internationalizing' of Cultural Studies", *Cultural Studies* 23(5), pp. 694–719.

SHOME, RAKA and HEGDE, RADHA (2002) "Postcolonial Approaches to Communication: charting the terrain, engaging the intersections", *Communication Theory* 12(3), pp. 249–70.

SOJA, EDWARD (1989) *Postmodern Geographies: the reassertion of space in critical social theory*, London: Verso.

SPARKS, COLIN (2000) "The Global, the Local and the Public Sphere", in: Gorgette Wang, Jan Servaes and Anura Goonasekera (Eds), *The New Communications Landscape: demystifying media globalization*, London: Routledge, pp. 74–95.

SPIVAK, GAYATRI CHAKRAVORTY (2003) *Death of a Discipline*, New York: Columbia University Press.

SPIVAK, GAYATRI CHAKRAVORTY (2008) *Other Asias*, Malden, MA: Blackwell Publishing.

STRAUBHAAR, JOSEPH (2007) *World Television: from global to local*, Newbury Park, CA: Sage.

THUSSU, DAYA (2006) *Media on the Move: global flow and contra-flow*, London: Taylor & Francis.

XIE, SHAOBO (2006) "Is the World Decentered? A postcolonialist perspective on globalization", in: Clara Joseph and Janet Wilson (Eds), *Global Fissures: postcolonial fusions*, Amsterdam: Rodopi, pp. 53–77.

YOUNG, ROBERT (2001) *Postcolonialism: an introduction*, London: Blackwell.

TOWARDS A GLOBAL JOURNALISM ETHICS VIA LOCAL NARRATIVES
Southern African perspectives

Herman Wasserman

This article argues that a global media ethics can only be arrived at via a study of local contexts. Following the notion of a "critical dialogic ethics" suggested by Christians, it is argued that a global media ethics should be constructed not as an overarching framework or global social contract arrived at through rational deliberation of ethical concepts removed from historical contexts, everyday lived experience and embedded practices, but through critical dialogue and interaction with Others within those contexts. An ethnographic, cultural approach that seeks narrative accounts of local values and practices should go beyond accepting local values and practices as unalterable or essentialist. Such a global dialogic ethics would start with thick descriptions of contextual values and practices. This article offers a first step towards a description of such values and practices within two particular African contexts, South Africa and Namibia. The contextual understanding of normative concepts of "social responsibility" and "freedom" are explored in journalistic narratives. The article points to conflicting interpretations of these notions and highlighting the need for an approach to global media ethics that takes account of the complexity of African contexts.

Introduction

One of the central questions in media ethics scholarship in recent years has been whether a global media ethics is possible, and what it could look like. One of the most challenging concerns in these debates (see, for instance, Black and Barney, 2002; Christians et al., 2008; Cooper et al., 1989; Wasserman, 2010a) has been how to account for a diversity of ethical perspectives globally, while avoiding cultural relativism. The incorporation of these various "local" perspectives into a global media ethic is further complicated by the fact that "local" or "regional" perspectives may themselves offer competing visions of what a "global" media ethics would look like, or even question whether such a global ethics is possible or desirable.

At first glance, media ethics codes globally agree, at least denotatively, on the centrality of concepts such as media freedom, truth-telling, independence and respon-sibility (Christians et al., 2008, p. 138). A particularly influential framework for thinking about how media should use its freedom to the benefit of society has been the social responsibility framework, originally developed in the United States by the Hutchins Commission in 1947. It has been suggested that this framework, despite its shortcomings and US-centred history, has "won global recognition" (Christians and Nordenstreng, 2004, p. 4), adopted in national media systems, and influenced debates about equitable global communication systems, such as those around the New World Information and

Communication Order at UNESCO in the late 1970s (Christians and Nordenstreng, 2004, p. 6). However, the wide adoption of the notion of social responsibility might obscure the fact that tensions between freedom and responsibility remain, even in established democracies, and that the framework's genesis in a particular historical and geographic context might make it an inadequate foundation for global media ethics. Hence Christians and Nordenstreng (2004) propose that global social responsibility should instead be based on universal proto-norms such as human dignity, truth-telling, and non-malfeasance.

Critical contributions from the perspective of postcolonial theory (Rao and Wasserman, 2007; Wasserman and Rao, 2008) have suggested that media ethical constructs such as freedom and responsibility, which are often presented as having universal validity, are themselves "local" in that they have originated from particular epistemological traditions rooted in Western thought and experience. These critics have argued that grand and totalizing schemes for global media ethics have to make way for more nuanced understandings of the specific cultural and political histories within which ethics are interpreted and operationalized, especially in various settings outside the Northern metropolitan centers. The very notion of universalism, with its historical association with the exercise of Western power, also needs to be examined critically (for a related critique of discourses of "internationalization" in the field of cultural studies, see Shome, 2009). Localized understandings of global norms are important in order to re-inscribe "Otherness" and difference into global media narratives. This introduction of non-Western perspectives into a "global" narrative needs to go beyond superficial and patronizing gestures of inclusion and diversity. A tokenistic inclusion of the Other as a way of validating the hegemony of existing, dominant frameworks may (albeit inadvertently) result in a relativistic ethics (where local ethical norms are merely included but not engaged critically).

The refusal to engage with the ethics of the Other on a deep theoretical level may result in a tacit validation of cultural norms that might be highly problematic (one thinks for instance of cultural claims around "dignity" and "respect" in African cultures that may be abused to prevent criticism of government). A superficial engagement of Other perspectives on media ethics (for instance as descriptive case studies to illustrate existing theoretical notions) may also render them exotic and static, ignoring the vigorous contestations around central moral concepts that take place in these localized contexts. While it is clear that simplistic notions of the "universal" will not do justice to the global cultural diversity reflected in different ethical norms, the "local" equally is not an unproblematic category through which to approach global media ethics either. It is true that regions outside the Global North—"Chindia", Southern Africa, the Middle East (with Rupert Murdoch recently announcing the establishment of the Middle East headquarters of News Corporation in Abu Dhabi) and South Asia (see Rao's paper in this issue: Rao, 2011)—necessitate new ways of looking at the global mediascape. Nation-based approaches to "international media" have to make way for "transnational" perspectives which acknowledge not only the emergence of influential regions, but also the increased diversity within nations of the global North, as induced by the rise of diasporic media. Within these regions and localities, significant contestation may exist between various ethical traditions.

This paper seeks to continue the critique of social responsibility and freedom as normative foundations for a global media ethic by exploring various interpretations of these within a region of the Global South, drawing on empirical data from two African countries—South Africa and Namibia. Apart from illustrating the specific negotiations and contestations around two central media ethical terms in these two countries, the article also models an approach to global ethics via the local that is rooted in narrative. Instead of a global media ethics based on social contract thinking, which might be based on the rational deliberation between interlocutors around ethical concepts, a narrative approach would seek to understand how ethical concepts are interpreted, applied and given meaning within specific, concrete, geo-historical contexts. Such an approach would be rooted in an ethnographic understanding of morality, that is, the realisation that "morality is rooted in everyday experience and gains multiple levels of complexity" (Christians, 2010, p. 178). The narrative approach would eschew the notion, based in Enlightenment thinking, that a global social contract for media ethics may be arrived at via arguments about the authority and validity of ethical rules and concepts in a rational and deliberative way. In a postmodern, fragmented global society, getting moral agents to participate in, let alone agree on, a formalist set of norms for global media, might be unattainable. Following MacIntyre, Christians (2010, p. 179) argues for a perspective on media ethics rooted in "the way humans actually experience life and how they interpret it, that is, in narrative". Moral action arises out of "our life narratives lived out in a historical context" (Christians, 2010, p. 179), and so a "shift from principle to story, from formal logic to community formation, is appealing" (2010, p. 180). Christians, linking also to James Carey's notion of "communication as culture", explains how narrative provides a path to moral understanding:

> Narratives are linguistic forms through which we argue, persuade, display convictions, and establish our identity. They contain in a nutshell the meaning of our theories and beliefs. We tell stories to one another about our values and concerns, and our aspirations. (Christians, 2010, p. 181)

Within the context of the search for global media ethics, such a dialogic approach that seeks to uncover the voices of the Other would, however, also have to include a critical dimension. In order to avoid cultural and moral relativism, the global dialogue should go beyond the mere inclusion of a diversity of voices to a critical dialogue that interrogates ethical traditions and understandings in terms of their adherence to the global proto-norms of human dignity, truth-telling, and non-malfeasance (Christians and Nordenstreng, 2004). If such a critical interrogation does not take place, a global narrative ethics might end up being a mere collection of ethical stories that remain unchallenged and perhaps incompatible. That way cultural essentialism and moral relativism lie. Instead, a global narrative ethics that simultaneously (1) takes global cultural diversity seriously rather than incorporate it as epistemological exotica, (2) avoids treating whole regions and traditions as homogenous and internally uncontested, and (3) refuses to acquiesce in claims to cultural essentialisms, will have to be truly dialogical *and* critical:

> A normative dialogic paradigm is a decisive alternative to relativism and a fruitful framework for communications in an age of globalization and multiculturalism. In formalist ethics, all acts are monologic, although actions may be coordinated with others. When humans are understood as cultural beings, however, human action is dialogic. (Christians, 2010, p. 183)

This article aims to make a modest beginning in the process of understanding media ethics within geographic and historic localities in such a narrative, dialogic way. It aims to highlight how ethical concepts (in this case "freedom" and "responsibility") are understood within specific contexts, how these understandings are coloured by history and influenced by politics and culture, and how the meanings journalists make out of these ethical concepts throw up a varied, textured and sometimes contested picture. This varied picture can enrich our understanding of global media ethics, by helping us see better how global ethical concepts are embodied, immersed and lived in localities. Before going on to a summary of the narratives obtained from journalists working in South Africa and Namibia, a brief overview of the context might be helpful.

Media Ethics in Africa

In the era of globalization, African media increasingly have to negotiate the space between ethical norms and practices as these have evolved in a particular socio-cultural and political environment, on the one hand, and globalized ethical discourses laying claim to universal validity, on the other hand. An example of the intersection between universal and regional discourses was the landmark Windhoek Declaration on Promoting an Independent and Pluralistic African Press in 1991 (Windhoek Declaration, 1991). In this declaration, African journalists invoked the Universal Declaration of Human Rights as a motivation for the promotion of press freedom in the particular African context. The spread of global media to African audiences (for instance, through satellite television) and the reach of African media to global audiences (for instance through new media technologies such as the Internet often aimed at Africans in the diaspora) have positioned African media ethics in a context that is increasingly transnational. For African media ethicists, this global–local intersection poses challenges. What norms should be used when evaluating media content in this transnational sphere? Are African ethical norms appropriate to deal with globalized media in a postmodern age? Conversely, can ethical frameworks derived from the Global North provide appropriate guidelines for ethical action in African contexts that differ in many respects from those in which dominant normative media theories have been devised?

As several case studies from Africa (e.g. Lodamo and Skjerdal, 2009; Ndangam, 2006) have made clear, the circumstances under which African journalists work are often so radically different from those in the North, that a wholesale importation of Northern ethical frameworks would be unsuitable for these conditions. More recent scholarly concerns with "global media ethics" run the risk of again (albeit inadvertently) imposing Northern norms under the guise of universalism, as postcolonial critics have argued (Rao and Wasserman, 2007; Wasserman, 2006). Perhaps the best-known African response to Northern ethics came from the Zambian ethicist Francis Kasoma (see Kasoma, 1994, 1996, 2000). His attempt to construct an Afri-ethics has, however, invited criticism for its romantic notions of an idyllic African society untouched by the West (e.g. Banda, 2009; Nyamnjoh, 2005, p. 91). Because of the dangers of essentializing African culture (cf. critique by Tomaselli, 2003) when African media practices are contrasted against Western norms, other scholars (e.g. Christians, 2004; Wasserman and De Beer, 2004) have sought connections between indigenous ethical frameworks such as *ubuntu* and Western approaches like communitarianism rather than pitting them against each other (Fourie, 2007).

Media ethics in Africa can, therefore, be seen as contested terrain. Various normative frameworks continue to co-exist and compete for dominance over media ethical discourses. These ethical frameworks also have a political dimension, as they may support conflicting visions of who African media owe their primary *responsibility* to, and what their degree of *freedom* should be. It should not be taken for granted that the use of central ethical concepts such as media freedom and social responsibility in African media contexts necessarily correspond with the way these terms are used elsewhere. Nor should it be assumed that these ethical values are understood in the same way across various African contexts or even between different sections of the media in African countries.

This article will proceed to summarize three of the main ethical frameworks (development journalism, indigenous ethics, and professionalization) that have been used in African media contexts, before going on to illustrate how these various frameworks continue to co-exist in the normative views of media practitioners today. Interview responses[1] from journalists in South Africa and Namibia were used to explore how journalists articulate their interpretation of the concepts of responsibility and freedom, and how these articulations relate to these broader frameworks. Journalists were asked to describe the way they see their role in relation to the public (their social responsibility) and towards the government (the degree of freedom they enjoy or think they should enjoy). The findings demonstrate how journalists in these African democracies negotiate their varying duties and loyalties, and how they balance obligation to freedom and responsibilities.

Development Journalism Framework

One of the defining normative frameworks within which journalists in Africa have understood their role has been that of development journalism. Although originating in Asia in the 1960s, the approach also gained popularity in Africa and Latin America (Xiaoge, 2009, p. 357), and as such may be seen as a transnational normative framework for developing regions (Christians et al., 2009, p. 200). Development journalism may be seen as an attempt to develop collaboration between media and governments into a normative theory (Christians et al., 2009, p. 198). Responsibility in this framework is articulated in terms of the media's role to promote development, which in practice has mostly meant supporting governments in attaining their economic, political, and cultural development goals. Often seen as antithetical to the Western libertarian approach, development journalism has indeed been vulnerable to abuse by postcolonial governments.

This is not to say that development journalism is incompatible with Western frameworks of social responsibility. When understood as a type of journalism that examines, evaluates, and reports on the relevance and success of development programs (also criticizing governments who fall short of developmental goals), development journalism can be consistent with the social responsibility theory (Ogan, 1982, p. 10), although arguably such a definition of development journalism might not be based on collaboration (Christians et al., 2009, pp. 198–9) anymore. An alternative notion of "emancipatory journalism" (Shah, 1996) has also been proposed as a way to redirect attention to the way journalism can affect social change and improve people's living conditions instead of focusing primarily on the relationship between media and the state.

Despite the problems inherent in development journalism as a normative framework, it continues to feature strongly in contemporary discourses of African journalism. As African journalism practices are increasingly infused with global philosophies and ideologies, and African media institutions are integrated into a globalized media landscape, African journalists have to balance globalized assumptions with the expectations and imperatives of the societies in the developing world within which they work (Musa and Domatob, 2007, p. 315). As a result, the role of journalists in developing countries is "complex, sometimes contradictory" (Musa and Domatob, 2007, p. 317). Within this framework, seemingly universal values such as freedom and responsibility might correspond notionally but are interpreted and operationalized differently. As Musa and Domatob state:

> At critical junctures, the fault lines in the perceived common ground between development journalists and their Western counterparts have been exposed. From the time of the anti-colonial struggles of the 1950s and 1960s to the post 9/11 world, it has become obvious that when First World and Third World journalists say they are committed to truth, freedom, and the common good, they each have different understandings of these concepts or pursue them through different means. (2007, p. 320)

Later in this paper I will illustrate how these varying interpretations of similar normative concepts play out in the South African and Namibian media environment.

Indigenization of Ethics

Moves to develop indigenous media ethics in Africa were not only related to the developmental discourse but also resulted from increasing political pluralism and concomitant liberalization of the media in the 1990s. The "third wave of democratization" which spread across the continent in the 1990s in many cases meant greater freedom for journalists, but also demanded of journalists to "take responsibility for their unethical actions instead of blaming them on government" (Kasoma, 1994, p. 3). Francis Kasoma's "Afri-ethics" (see Banda, 2009 for a recent summary and re-assessment) was developed in an attempt to develop an ethical framework based on a strong sense of (religious) morality and communal bonds. For Kasoma, the increased media freedom as a result of media liberalization raised the imperative of greater responsibility towards African cultural and societal values:

> The urge to imitate the Americans and Europeans who introduced journalism into Africa—together with colonialism ... and evangelism—seems to have had much more influence on African journalists, than any sense of what would be appropriate, and right, in their own context. (Kasoma, 1994, p. 4)

Ethical actions "should take into account the African approach to life" even if it does choose to include principles and values from elsewhere (Kasoma, 1994, p. 8). These values should take into account the material conditions within which African journalists work (e.g. poor pay that make them susceptible to bribes; Kasoma, 1994, p. 19) but also the orientation towards the "family, clan and community" rather than towards the individual. This responsibility towards society in a communal sense rather than society as a collection of individuals distinguishes African ethics from Western approaches (Kasoma, 1994, p. 27). In such a communal orientation, consensus is seen as more important than a majority or utilitarian decision (Kasoma, 1994, p. 28). Although Kasoma points out that consensus should not be mistaken for the uncritical support of national unity as imposed by governments, Tomaselli (2003, p. 430) has characterized Kasoma's view of the media as being more of a "guidedog" than a "watchdog".

In recent years, especially after the end of apartheid in South Africa, renewed attempts have been made to rediscover idealized values of African culture. An example is the relational African philosophy of *ubuntu* in South Africa, which can be summed up "I am because you are" (Christians, 2004; Wasserman and De Beer, 2004). Critics (Banda, 2009; Fourie, 2007; Tomaselli, 2003) have, however, warned that attempts to construct or re-validate an African ethics may pose several dangers. Among these are the danger of cultural essentialism and cultural exceptionalism which sets African ethics apart from outside critique and serves the interests of an elite-class prescriptive and generalized discourse of pan-African values (Tomaselli, 2003, p. 430). Attempts to indigenize ethics often treats Africa as a monolith, glossing over complex social and cultural differences and presenting African culture in romantic, idealized terms, with little acknowledgement of how African cultures have been influenced by historical processes such as colonialism, nationalism, and globalization (Banda, 2009, p. 236; Tomaselli, 2009, p. 13). The resurrection of idealized African values moreover does not take into account the contemporary African media's location in a globalizing world and a changing media environment, where diversity and pluralism, rather than static cultural norms, are valued (Fourie, 2007). Using "African values" as a normative basis for media practice is also seen as posing a threat to freedom of expression because criticism of government or politicians may be cast as un-African, un-patriotic, or disrespectful towards authority (Fourie, 2007; Tomaselli, 2009, p. 13).

As Banda (2009) has argued, the pitfalls of indigenous African ethics do not necessarily preclude the possibility of developing an ethical framework more attuned to African social and cultural values. A reappraisal of African ethics would, however, need to incorporate democratic citizenship and empowerment (Banda, 2009) in order for it to be applicable. Such a reappraisal would also require a new definition of culture (Tomaselli, 2009, p. 11) which moves away from anthropological notions of African culture as bounded ways of life, culture as high/low in aesthetic terms or social behaviour, in order to position African media content and audiences in terms of globalizing cultural flows and fragmented, dynamic cultural difference. In a postmodern global media landscape, marked by complex transnational cultural flows, commonly held notions of Africanness are fractured (Tomaselli, 2009, p. 15), and a normative framework based on homogenous cultural values or populist calls for a return to tradition becomes untenable.

Professionalism and Social Responsibility

The realization that networks of meaning and social identities in African societies are experiencing rapid transitions as a result of global cultural flows (Tomaselli, 2009, p. 16), have led to calls for more dynamic ways of envisaging the relationship between freedom and responsibility. Under the influence of global narratives of media freedom, journalistic professionalism and democratic participation, central values for media ethics in con-temporary Africa are being linked to the importance of critique as a feature of robust democracy, the opening up of spaces for debate and the inclusion of a plurality of voices and participation in a global dialogue (Tomaselli, 2009, p. 17).

The interventionist strategies of "media development", driven by non-governmental organizations and funding bodies in the North with an aim of capacitating media in the South, can be seen as part of this trend (Berger, 2010). Underpinning the capacity-building activities of these organizations in Africa is the normative assumption that vibrant media will lead to more democratic societies—"media development" therefore becomes "subject to particular cultural and even political preferences" (Berger, 2010, p. 552). The "political preference" of non-state actors involved in the promotion of media ethics in Africa ("through conference, workshops and symposia"; Mfumbusa, 2008, p. 143) has more often than not been inclined towards liberalism, seeing the media as linked to individual rights and a free-market environment, and encouraging the professionalization of journalism.

These codes developed for African democracies (e.g. in South Africa) are frequently influenced by notions of freedom and social responsibility derived from the Global North (see Retief, 2002, p. 20; Wasserman, 2006). These values sometimes conflict with prevailing cultural norms, and the failure of African journalists to comply with these professional standards and norms are often lamented (Mfumbusa, 2008, pp. 141–2). Notions of "freedom" and "responsibility" are therefore contested within African media contexts, as we will see in more detail below.

Freedom and Responsibility in the South African and Namibian Context

White (2010) argues for an empirical approach to normative ethics in Africa that takes its starting point not in theoretical abstractions but in an observation of journalists' reasoning. This approach advocated by White would correspond with the narrative or critical dialogical approach to media ethics described above. Going about in this way may help to establish what motivates journalists in Africa and how they view their role in relation to society. From an analysis of media practice, the underlying normative perspectives of these practices may then be established. The findings of this study draw on interviews with South African and Namibian journalists in which they were asked to explain how they see their role in society and how they understand the concepts of freedom and responsibility. These interviews have been conducted within the context of South Africa and Namibia as new democracies emerging from a period of authoritarian rule by the apartheid regime in South Africa and South Africa's occupation of Namibia. (Some of this data has also been used more extensively in Wasserman, 2010b, within the broader context of political journalism in transitional democracies). The comparative study sought to uncover the various discourses through which journalists give meaning to central ethical concepts and how conflicting interpretations of freedom and responsibility might arise out of these various discourses.

Media Freedom

Respondents were asked to assess the level of media freedom in their countries and to identify threats posed to that freedom. In the course of this assessment, definitions also emerged of what "freedom" means in the context of African democracies.

In South Africa, several direct threats to media freedom were identified, e.g. the ruling ANC's proposal that a Media Tribunal be established to replace the self-regulation by the Press Ombudsman (see Duncan, 2010). More subtle political threats included perceived government influence in the editorial content of the public broadcaster, the South African Broadcasting Corporation, and the appointment of its Board. From responses of journalists it became clear that any intervention from the government into professional journalistic practices is being strongly resisted. The collaboration between media and government proposed in the developmental journalism framework is widely rejected by media practitioners who value freedom as the cornerstone of their professional ethics. As will be seen in the responses quoted below, the notion of "responsibility" is often seen as a threat to that freedom.

In Namibia, concerns were also expressed about political threats emerging in the post-independence period. Intermediaries remarked on the government's sensitivity to criticism; journalists reported intimidation and were "becoming more and more worried" that they had to be "very, very much careful about what you say". One recurring fear was the government's threat to establish a Media Council to regulate media content (similar to the Media Tribunal proposed in South Africa, see Duncan, 2011). The remedy suggested by journalists was to establish a more vigorous system of self-regulation in line with normative values of independence and a watchdog function. This response from journalists points to the belief that an adherence to the professional and social responsibility framework with self-designed ethical codes will function as a safeguard against interference from government.

Namibian journalists pointed to the demand from government that the media should work with the government rather than against it as a thinly veiled attempt to silence critics. The appeal by the Namibian government is said often to be phrased in terms of respect for indigenous values, not unlike past calls by critics of the media in South Africa calling for a more African orientation in media reporting (e.g. Mbeki, 2003). These journalists found the indigenization of ethics or development journalism frameworks coming into conflict with their own views on professionalization and social responsibility. Namibian journalists complained that media criticism is often constructed as undermining of the good order in society and counter-democratic. One journalist summed it up:

> I will say in Namibia but also in the whole of the region especially is the tendency of people in power to sort of talk down to the media . . . to portray criticism as unpatriotic, as a conspiracy . . . I think if you succeed . . . to diminish the role or the credibility of media from an official platform that . . . is a big threat to media freedom because if people think that they cannot take media seriously, they won't.

In both countries, economic threats to media freedom were also mentioned. The end of apartheid brought a shift towards increased commercialization of the South African media, as old ideological ties between media and political parties were severed and media entered a competitive global market-place. The attendant "juniorization" (laying off of senior staff and employing younger ones) and the dwindling of investigative or informative political reporting were among the most prominent themes that emerged from responses about new threats to press freedom. Commercialization was seen as leading to self-censorship and "dumbing down" of content. Journalists remarked on how increasing commercial pressures made it difficult for them to pursue investigative or in-depth projects.

In Namibia, the commercialization of the media was also seen as a threat to freedom. A particular sticking point was the use of tax money to fund the state-owned newspaper, which was described, by one journalist, as "giving your enemy bullets". This strong opposition to government-ownership of the media reiterates the high value attached to media freedom by journalists, and makes it unlikely that the indigenization or developmental frameworks of media ethics, usually supported (at least rhetorically) by the media's political opponents, will gain acceptance among journalists.

The fact that journalists not only remarked on politically-motivated threats to freedom but also expressed concern about commercial pressures eroding their ability to conduct investigative journalism suggests that media freedom was frequently seen as linked to social responsibility, rather than viewed as an absolute value. But what exactly responsibility entails was also reason for disagreement.

Media Responsibility

In both the countries two conflicting positions came to the fore regarding media responsibility. It was either seen as linked to democratic freedom, so that certain restraints were in order (in terms of the social responsibility approach), or it was viewed with suspicion by journalists as an excuse for governments to exercise control over media content (often by making rhetorical claims to the developmental journalism or indigenization frameworks). The difference between these two attitudes can be linked to normative emphases on either independence and freedom or social responsibility.

Firstly, among those journalists who saw responsibility as a corollary of freedom, there were mixed opinions as to whether the media succeeds in acting responsibly. Some of the general terms associated with media responsibility were "transparency", "account-ability", "accuracy", people's "dignity and reputation", the avoidance of incitement to violence and harm or "the fact that you cannot extend your freedom to harm another". Rooting out corruption and speaking out for the voiceless were also seen as hallmarks of responsibility.

Some journalists were, however, more open to self-criticism and acknowledged the need for some restraint. One said: "I think that (responsibility) is also to address those issues when we abuse that freedom ... Media freedom comes with a hell of a responsibility". Understandably, in the light of South Africa's history, stereotyping, especially regarding racism and xenophobia, were singled out by a number of respondents as an area where restraint on press freedom was deemed necessary.

Where journalists described this restraint in terms such as "protection of (human) rights" or the "social well-being of a community", their views displayed similarities with the indigenization discourse, where ethical responsibilities are seen as being owed to an interrelated community rather than to a collection of individuals (cf. the discussion of *ubuntu* above). The notions of "dignity" and "respect" may also be a response to South Africa's history of human rights abuses, against which the media did not always provide enough resistance. Consequently, journalists often defined "responsibility" in terms of an adversarial stance against current governments in South Africa and Namibia.

Journalists, however, often resisted the very notion of "responsibility" as a potential strategy for governments to restrict media freedom. Journalists seemed to be aware of the possibility that those in power may abuse especially the development and indigenization discourses to force the media to adhere to a narrow notion of "responsibility"—one which means more or less the same as loyalty to the government. Journalists adhering to this view rejected any notion of "responsibility" as representative of a political agenda. Conversely, some journalists saw such resistance to governmental interference as precisely their "responsibility". For these respondents the media in these two countries had the responsibility of acting almost as the unofficial political opposition.

Conclusion

A global media ethic would have to include perspectives from Africa. African media ethics can, however, by no means be seen as an homogenous area. Media ethics in Africa remain a contested terrain with media ethics scholars drawing on divergent frameworks to argue for the optimal relation between media freedom and media responsibility in African democracies. This article identified the most prominent of these frameworks as the development journalism approach, the indigenization approach, and the professiona-lization and social responsibility approach. While the literature on media ethics in Africa has sometimes pitted Northern-influenced frameworks of social responsibility and individualistic notions of freedom against indigenous approaches (e.g. Kasoma, 1996), other scholars suggested that affinities may be found between indigenous African philosophies and Northern approaches like communitarianism (e.g. Christians, 2004), or that the social responsibility concept might be accommodated within a broader framework of development journalism (e.g. Ogan, 1982). The South African and Namibian journalists interviewed for this study, however, largely viewed these frameworks as oppositional; the notions of freedom and responsibility were at times contextualized to fit the particular democratic contexts. The development journalism and indigenization frameworks were largely viewed with suspicion as vehicles for new and subtle forms of pressure on freedom of speech in the two new countries. In everyday journalistic practice ethics is an outcome of a process of negotiation between stakeholders in the media and their counterparts in the political sphere.

What are the implications of these findings for the search for global media ethics? This contestation of normative frameworks suggests that it is impossible to speak of "African", "regional" or "local" ethics in any broad or monolithic manner. Historical and contemporary political, social and cultural factors impact on how ethical frameworks are adopted and operationalized. Furthermore, the negotiation of ethical frameworks takes place not only internally in African countries but is also linked to cultural flows and contra-flows between Africa and the rest of the world in a globalized media landscape. Influences from Northern media ethics are adopted, adapted and resisted in local contexts, and take on new social and political meanings. These complex processes fragment any simple or monolithic understanding of African ethics.

A global media ethics that seeks to incorporate perspectives from Africa would need to be cognizant of the full complexity of media ethics on this continent and in its various countries and regions, as well as how media ethics are operationalized and interpreted in everyday journalistic practice. Dealing with high-level concepts, or romanticized, essentialized notions of "African ethics" will not be helpful in arriving at a global ethics that includes Africa. Instead, a narrative approach that draws out the meaning-making processes around ethical concepts, in order to then engage in a critical dialogue with these ethical meanings, would be a much more fruitful approach. Such an approach calls for a more ethnographic and empirical approach to media ethics, one which would seek to first assess the attitudes and norms currently being negotiated in African settings but which then sets out to explore how these attitudes and norms articulate with various other ethical narratives in media settings in other parts of the world. Such a process would be a dynamic and open-ended one that refuses to reify Africa as a static repository of indigenous knowledge ready to be appropriated in global discourses, but rather as a terrain on which various ethical traditions and discourses continue to play out.

NOTE

1. These interviews formed part of a larger, comparative transnational study on political communication in new democracies, funded by the British Academy (LRG-45511), which covered: Southern Africa (Namibia, South Africa), East Asia (Taiwan, South Korea), Eastern Europe (Bulgaria, Poland) and Latin America (Brazil, Chile). Between eight and ten journalists were interviewed in each of these countries, in addition to interviews with politicians and intermediaries.

REFERENCES

BANDA, FACKSON (2009) "Kasoma's Afriethics: a reappraisal", *International Communication Gazette* 71(4), pp. 227–42.

BERGER, GUY (2010) "Problematizing 'Media Development' as a Bandwagon Gets Rolling", *International Communication Gazette* 72(7), pp. 547–65.

BLACK, JAY and BARNEY, RALPH (Eds) (2002) "Search for a Global Media Ethic" [Special Issue], *Journal of Mass Media Ethics* 17(4).

CHRISTIANS, CLIFFORD (2004) "Ubuntu and Communitarianism in Media Ethics", *Ecquid Novi: African Journalism Studies* 25(2), pp. 235–56.

CHRISTIANS, CLIFFORD (2010) "Communication Ethics in Postnarrative Terms", in: Linda Steiner and Clifford Christians (Eds), *Key Concepts in Critical Cultural Studies*, Urbana: University of Illinois Press, pp. 173–86.

CHRISTIANS, CLIFFORD and NORDENSTRENG, KAARLE (2004) "Social Responsibility Worldwide", *Journal of Mass Media Ethics* 19(1), pp. 3–28.

CHRISTIANS, CLIFFORD, RAO, SHAKUNTALA, WARD, STEPHEN J. and WASSERMAN, HERMAN (2008) "Toward a Global Media Ethics: exploring new theoretical perspectives", *Ecquid Novi: African Journalism Studies* 29(2), pp. 135–72.

CHRISTIANS, CLIFFORD G., GLASSER, THEODORE L., MCQUAIL, DENIS, NORDENSTRENG, KAARLE and WHITE, ROBERT A. (2009) *Normative Theories of the Media: Journalism in Democratic Societies*, Urbana and Chicago: University of Illinois Press.

COOPER, THOMAS W., CHRISTIANS, CLIFFORD G., PLUDE, FRANCES F. and WHITE, ROBERT A. (Eds) (1989) *Communication Ethics and Global Change*, White Plains, NY: Longman.

DUNCAN, JANE (2010) "The ANC's Poverty of Strategy on Media Accountability", *Ecquid Novi: African Journalism Studies* 31(2), pp. 90–105.

FOURIE, PIETER J. (2007) "Moral Philosophy as a Threat to Freedom of Expression: from Christian-Nationalism to *ubuntuism* as a normative framework for media regulation and practice in South Africa", *Communications—European Journal of Communication Research* 32, pp. 1–29.

KASOMA, FRANCIS P. (Ed.) (1994) *Journalism Ethics in Africa*, Nairobi: ACCE.

KASOMA, FRANCIS P. (1996) "The Foundations of African Ethics (Afriethics) and the Professional Practice of Journalism: the case for society-centred media morality", *Africa Media Review* 10(3), pp. 93–116.

KASOMA, FRANCIS P. (2000) *The Press and Multiparty Politics in Africa*, Tampere: University of Tampere.

LODAMO, BERHANU and SKJERDAL, TERJE S. (2009) "Freebies and Brown Envelopes in Ethiopian Journalism", *Ecquid Novi: African Journalism Studies* 30(2), pp. 134–54.

MBEKI, THABO (2003) "Address by the President of South Africa", address to the Sanef Conference on the Media, The AU, NEPAD and Democracy, Johannesburg, 12 April, http://www.info.gov.za/speeches/2003/03041410461001.htm, accessed 15 November 2010.

MFUMBUSA, BERNADIN F. (2008) "Newsroom Ethics in Africa: quest for a normative framework", *African Communication Research* 1(2), pp. 139–58.

MUSA, BALA and DOMATOB, JERRY K. (2007) "Who Is a Development Journalist? Perspectives on media ethics and professionalism in post-colonial societies", *Journal of Mass Media Ethics* 22(4), pp. 315–31.

NDANGAM, LILIAN (2006) "'Gombo': bribery and the corruption of journalism ethics in Cameroon", *Ecquid Novi: African Journalism Studies* 27(2), pp. 179–99.

NYAMNJOH, FRANCIS B. (2005) *Africa's Media—democracy and the politics of belonging*, London: Zed Books.

OGAN, CHRISTINE (1982) "Development Journalism/Communication: the status of the concept", *International Communication Gazette* 29(1/2), pp. 3–9.

RAO, SHAKUNTALA (2011) "The 'Local' in Global Media Ethics", *Journalism Studies* 12(6), pp. 780–90.

RAO, SHAKUNTALA and WASSERMAN, HERMAN (2007) "Global Journalism Ethics Revisited: a postcolonial critique", *Global Media and Communication* 3(1), pp. 29–50.

RETIEF, JOHAN (2002) *Media Ethics: an introduction to responsible journalism*, Cape Town: Oxford University Press.

SHAH, HEMANT (1996) "Modernization, Marginalization, and Emancipation: toward a normative model of journalism and national development", *Communication Theory* 6(2), pp. 143–66.

SHOME, RAKA (2009) "Post-colonial Reflections on the 'Internationalization' of Cultural Studies", *Cultural Studies* 23(5/6), pp. 694–719.

TOMASELLI, KEYAN G. (2003) "'Our Culture' vs. 'Foreign Culture': an essay on ontological and professional issues in African journalism", *Gazette* 65(6), pp. 427–41.

TOMASELLI, KEYAN G. (2009) "Repositioning African Media Studies: thoughts and provocations", *Journal of African Media Studies* 1(1), pp. 9–21.

WASSERMAN, HERMAN (2006) "Globalised Values and Postcolonial Responses: South African perspectives on normative media ethics", *The International Communication Gazette* 68(1), pp. 71–91.

WASSERMAN, HERMAN (2010a) "The Search for Global Journalism Ethics", in: C. Meyers (Ed.), *Philosophical Approaches to Journalism Ethics*, Oxford: Oxford University Press, pp. 69–84.

WASSERMAN, HERMAN (2010b) "Freedom's Just Another Word? Perspectives on the media freedom and responsibility in South Africa and Namibia", *International Communication Gazette* 72(7), pp. 567–88.

WASSERMAN, HERMAN and DE BEER, ARNOLD S. (2004) "Covering HIV/Aids: towards a heuristic comparison between communitarian and utilitarian ethics", *Communicatio* 30(2), pp. 84–97.

WASSERMAN, HERMAN and RAO, SHAKUNTALA (2008) "The Glocalization of Journalism Ethics", *Journalism: Theory, Practice Criticism* 9(2), pp. 163–81.

WHITE, ROBERT A. (2010) "The Moral Foundations of Media Ethics in Africa", *Ecquid Novi: African Journalism Studies* 31(1), pp. 42–67.

WINDHOEK DECLARATION (1991) "Windhoek Declaration on Promoting an Independent and Pluralistic African Press", www.chr.up.ac.za/hr_docs/african/docs/other/other23.doc, accessed 10 March 2010

XIAOGE, XU (2009) "Development Journalism", in: K. Wahl-Jorgensen and T. Hanitzsch (Eds), *The Handbook of Journalism Studies*, New York and Oxford: Routledge, pp. 357–70.

JOURNALISM'S MORAL SENTIMENTS
Negotiating between freedom and responsibility

Lee Wilkins

Philosophers since Adam Smith and David Hume have theorized that emotions play a role in ethical decision making. The most recent findings in neuroscience suggest that moral action does not occur without a firm handshake with the emotions. This paper explores the connection between emotions, bounded rationality and professional ethical decision making, specifically journalistic negotiation between freedom and responsibility. Based on the findings of neuroscience and coupled with feminist ethics and the concept of proto-norms as outlined by Christians, journalists' moral sentiments regarding these core concepts are linked to the development of a moral imagination that seeks both professionally sound and morally creative alternatives to difficult ethical choices. A case study of one documentary film maker illustrates the theory.

Overview

This paper is a second step along a path to integrate current findings in neuroscience with professional, specifically journalistic, ethics. As such, it attempts to answer the following question: How does professional ethical behavior—moral action—negotiate between two of the profession's most central philosophical tenants: freedom and responsibility? Current literature in the field tends to place these concepts at opposite ends of an Aristotelian continuum.

The theoretically based answer to this question focuses on two subsets of scholarly literature, current findings in neuroscience, specifically the concepts of bounded rationality and empathy, and the concepts of freedom and responsibility as they are understood philosophically and professionally. Then, feminist ethics and the concept of proto-norms, which have both rational and emotional components, are used to bridge these two bodies of literature and to suggest professional application. In particular, the approach is employed to explain ethical exemplars, professionals with an engaged moral imagination doing professionally and ethically excellent work. A brief case study of one documentary film maker is used to illustrate the major points and to suggest areas for further exploration.

The Evolution of a Debate

Earlier scholarship (Wilkins, 2008) has suggested the following framework for understanding moral behavior:

$$MB = (f)OE$$

where moral behavior is the function of a dynamic human organism within an environment. The human organism is dynamic; the recent findings of neuroscience suggest that human beings are "hard wired" to consider the ethical dimensions of intellectual questions (Gazzaniga, 2005; Hauser, 2006) and behavioral choices in much the same way that all human beings are hard wired to acquire language—although the specific languages they speak vary widely. Without repeating the entirety of the earlier argument, there is mounting evidence that, when it comes to many activities including moral behavior, human beings employ a mind-enhanced brain. The field of moral development (Kohlberg, 1981, 1984; Piaget, 1965; Rest, 1986; Rest et al., 1999) is closely intellectually and empirically connected to this understanding.

A central element characteristic of the mind-enhanced brain is the influence of emotion on cognitive processes. And, this is where disciplinary understandings begin to cloud the picture.

For traditional Enlightenment philosophers, beginning certainly with Descartes but extending through Kant and much of the contemporary era, rationality was both necessary and sufficient for ethical action. "Conceptual rationalism is committed to the claim that it is a conceptual truth that people who make moral judgments are motivated by them" (Nichols, 2004, p. 72). This reliance on rationality worked in tandem with a principle-based and top-down approach to ethical thinking, one that produced important insights about moral philosophy that focused on human virtues, duty and consequences. In the analysis required to understand these crucial paradigms of ethics, logic and rationality were intended to supersede the emotions, which were viewed as an impediment to rational thinking and subsequently to appropriate moral behavior.

Yet, some philosophers suggested a role for the emotions. Hume phrased it this way,

> The final sentence, it is probable, which pronounces characters and actions amiable or odious, praise-worthy or blameable; . . . that which renders morality an active principle . . . depends on some internal sense or feeling, which nature has made university in the whole species. For what else can have an influence of this nature? (1975 [1777], p. 173)

Adam Smith, the philosopher who first used the phrase "moral sentiments" (2010 [1759]), also did not discard the emotions. The potential for universal applicability of linking emotion and ethics was never fully explored by either, perhaps because many human emotions seem to fund violence and aggression, which often led to horrific and certainly unethical relations among human beings. The insights of Smith and Hume were generally less influential than those founded more in the exclusively rational approach, particularly in their contributions to philosophy and specifically meta-ethics. In the early twentieth century, the approaches recalling Smith and Hume were called either sentimentalism or emotivism. In some instances, they were also linked with intuitionism (Audi, 2005). Regardless, "the central challenge for sentimentalism is to preserve the idea that values are somehow grounded in the sentiments, while, at the same time making sense of the rational aspects of evaluation" (D'Arms and Jacobson, 2000, p. 722).

Although sentimentalism had a well-understood philosophical challenge, putting equal pressure on rationality was not taken up by philosophers who, in the main, eschewed empirical testing for continued theory building which sometimes relied on the device of "thought problems" without ever subjecting those same problems to real-world evaluation. That initial test of the concept, somewhat ironically, emerged from the discipline that Adam Smith is credited with founding: economics. Economic theory accepted the rational human actor as bedrock, but because the discipline deals with the "real world" it was inevitable that real-world decisions would be compared with this pre-eminent rationalism. In 1983, economist Herbert A. Simon coined the term "bounded rationality" to explain actual economic decision making. Based on empirical work, Simon initiated what has become a paradigm shift by noting,

> In this essay, I will focus initially on the very powerful formal models of rationality that have been constructed in this century and that must be counted among the jewels of intellectual accomplishment in our time. Since these models are well known, I will describe them only briefly, devoting most of my discussion to showing why, in application to real human affairs, they deliver somewhat less than they appear to promise. But, my intent here is not mainly critical. The last half of this [essay] will develop a more realistic description of human bounded rationality, and will consider to what extent the limited capability for analysis that is provided by bounded rationality can meet the needs for reason in human affairs ... (Simon in Moser, 1990, p. 189)

From this strong intellectual claim supported by substantial evidence, the concepts of decision making under uncertainty, of risk perception and decision making, and the sub-discipline of experimental economics emerged, all claiming the psychological processes were every bit as important to human decision making as rational, rule-based approaches (see, for example, Moser, 1990).

Emotions, of course, are the realm of the discipline of psychology, and while Simon coined the term bounded rationality, psychologists investigated how emotions influenced, sometimes profoundly, human decision making. As research methods became more sophisticated, it was possible to document that emotion employed different pathways in the brain, that emotion often preceded other sorts of cognitive activities, including logic— although preceded was often a matter of nanoseconds—and that human perception and thought was subject to predictable biases that appeared to trump rationality regardless of outcome. "This neurophysiological evidence gives rise to opposing views about how emotions and cognitions interact to influence decision making. Some argue strongly that there are two separate, independent systems for making decisions; while others argue that these two sources are integrated into a single emotional-cognitive decision-making process (Busemeyer et al., 2007, p. 215). "A single integrated system approach has been advocated by a smaller number of theorists. According to this view, emotions provide dynamic signals that feed into and help guide the cognitive system over time for making decisions ... Decision field theory provides dynamic mechanisms for integrating fast emotional signals with slower cognition information to guide decision making" (Busemeyer et al., 2007, p. 216). Scholarly study of journalists suggests that the use of emotions as dynamic signals in professional decision making is an appropriate view of the joint workings of emotion and cognition (Coleman and Wilkins, 2002, 2004; Wilkins and Coleman, 2005).

As if things had not become intellectually complicated enough, there was yet one more major intellectual stream that contributed to the river of often contentious empirical work on the nature of the human mind contained within the anatomical brain: evolutionary biology. Darwin, too, had written about a human "moral organ", and biologists, in their efforts to understand the species, began to discover and document the ability of many species, but particularly the higher apes, to engage in what looked like moral behavior (or its precursors) in humans (De Waal, 1996). "Altruism, compassion, empathy, love, conscience, the sense of justice—all of these things, the things that hold society together, the things that allow our species to think so highly of itself, can now confidently be said to have a firm genetic basis. That's the good news. The bad news is that although these things are in some ways blessings for humanity as a whole, they did not evolve for the 'good of the species' and are not reliably employed to that end. Quite the contrary, it is now clearer than ever (and precisely why) the moral sentiments are used with brutal flexibility, switching on and off in keeping with self-interest; and how naturally oblivious we often are to this switching. In the new view, human beings are a species splendid in their moral equipment, tragic in their propensity to misuse it, and pathetic in their constitutional ignorance of its misuse" (Wright, 1994, pp. 12–13).

So, at the beginning of this century at least three disciplines, philosophy, psychology, and evolutionary biology, had begun to devote considerable intellectual energy to understanding, theoretically and practically, how human beings make moral choices and what the results of those choices ought be. This convergence of intellectual energy suggests the following core understandings:

1. That human beings are demonstrably imperfectly rational. As a species, we seem to share this with our biological forebears.
2. That emotion (the moral sentiments) has a significant impact on moral choice, hence bounding and sustaining human rationality.
3. That how human beings think about morality and ethics is hard wired into the human mind-enhanced brain, where it co-exists with hard wiring about language and emotion, among other important things.
4. That thinking about ethics must account for empirical findings; as such, it must move beyond Enlightenment framing of questions without abandoning hard-won under-standings.

Within this emerging framework, professional ethics must seek its own intellectual ground. It is to that effort that this paper now turns.

Professional Freedom and Responsibility

Freedom and responsibility are difficult concepts with an ancient lineage. When journalists use the words, they most often mean them within the context of an institu-tional role: the duties, obligations and opportunities of journalists and the organizations for which they work within political society. In the recent history of the term, political society most often means democratic society. Thus journalists, individually and collectively, are both free and responsible to keep and maintain democratic commitments. They inhabit one institution among many. In the American context, professional journalistic freedom may result in other individuals or other institutions being made less free or held morally accountable for acts and their consequences. Journalists, individually and collectively, are also held morally accountable through a system of laws, at least in contemporary society, although there is huge debate about the degree of accountability particular societies achieve. One of the most important areas of current professional debate is whether journalists and journalism have this same role responsibility outside of a democratic context. The foregoing summarizes the dominant professional paradigm.

Such a conceptualization slides over a number of important philosophical debates. To begin with, philosophers starting with Aristotle (1999) have held individuals responsible for their acts. The fact that individuals could be held responsible suggested that they were free to act in multiple ways. This line of logic has resulted in what philosophers term moral agency, translated into contemporary thinking as the "autonomous moral actor". This is what Hume, and many others, meant when they used the words "praiseworthy" or "blameworthy" to evaluate ethical choice; praise or blame adheres to individuals acting on their own volition. These conceptualizations do have an emotional as well as a rational component. The range of potential actions available to the autonomous moral actor, in turn, raised questions of free will—if individuals were constrained from acting in specific ways, they could not then be held responsible for actions they had no power to make or to avoid. It is, therefore, not surprising that one of the objections to the notion of the human mind-enhanced brain being "hard wired" for fair (Hauser, 2006) is that such a construct seems, at least superficially, to challenge any notion of free will and hence of autonomous moral action. Without going into the debate in detail, most neuroscientists interpret their data as indicating that the brain-enhanced mind does not predispose human beings to act in any specific way when making moral decisions; a wide range of options, most certainly including immoral actions, remain open to people. These findings emerge from studies on "normal" human beings as well as those with traumatic brain injury and psychopaths. Although empirical findings do not constitute a complete rebuttal to the objection, they do suggest that moral agency remains a viable concept both for philosophy and for neuroscientists studying how people respond to ethical dilemmas. People appear to have vast freedom of choice; not everyone provides the same answer to the "trolley problem" and its many permutations.

Philosophical thinking since the Enlightenment has added some additional layers to the concept. John Stuart Mill, in his political tract "On Liberty" (1859), connected freedom to consequences of acts on the community. The social contract theorists, specifically Hobbes, Locke and Rousseau, espoused both a positive construction of liberty—freedom to form community—and a negative one—freedom from, specifically freedom from government intervention with individual acts within a community. Hobbes, particularly in his description of political life outside the social contract, assumes an emotional as well as rational motivation for individuals to leave the state of nature. Since modern understandings of the role of Western journalism (Ward, 2004) emerge from this era, it is not surprising that freedom from government intervention takes such a predominant role in the discussion of press freedom in the United States and Europe. In fact, some scholars such as Merrill (1974) see freedom from external constraint as the single most important ethical virtue for journalists as individuals and journalism in its democratic role. Merrill's particular construction emphasizes the individual over the community, a break with political philosophy of the seventeenth and eighteenth centuries, but one that has received wide notice and considerable acceptance in the twentieth century. In this view, freedom and responsibility are dichotomous.

With this political and social history, it is responsibility that becomes problematic. If journalists represent the institution that holds others to account, what institution can perform that same function for the media? The United States emphatically and constitutionally has rejected a role for the central government in such apportioning of responsibility; even nations without a written constitution, for example many in western Europe, have come to essentially the same political conclusions through the working out of history and precedent. Furthermore, because journalism is no longer in the day of the pamphleteer (although bloggers may be a close parallel), individual acts are not the only problem. How does one hold institutions responsible, produce what philosophers term collective responsibility? This is particularly difficult in the United States, where individual journalistic actions enjoy wide constitutional latitude and collective responsibility is often shunted to the market or to public condemnation, both ill-timed and imperfect forms of feedback and constraint. Communitarian philosophy, particularly a call for journalism that emerges from community and is responsive and responsible to it, has been the most prominent academic answer to the tension between freedom and responsibility. Communitarian journalism is transformational in nature; it employs justice as the mediating virtue (Christians et al., 1993). Communitarianism takes collective responsibility seriously; enforcement, either on the individual or institutional level, is less clearly articulated other than through moral suasion.

Finally, both freedom and responsibility carry emotional weight (Rao and Lee, 2005; Wilkins and Coleman, 2005). This is particularly true for individual journalists, regardless of country or origin. Twentieth-century history is replete with examples of journalist in many cultures and many political systems overcoming external constraints on their professional role. This effort is not bloodless, in either the literal or the metaphorical sense. Regardless of culture, these journalists are viewed as moral exemplars. They embody freedom, but they are also responsible to professional ideals that link to human virtue. They are free to be responsible to themselves and to others in particular societies and culture. How other professionals, and the scholars who study them, might understand their acts is the next step in the process.

Professional Rationality: Bounded and Supported by Emotional Commitments

The foregoing review is meant, at the most abstract level, to illustrate why dichotomies are sometimes less than helpful in moving the project of building theory forward. For most of the last 3000 years, academic and professional philosophy has struggled with what evidence suggests is a false dichotomy—reason or emotion. In much more recent professional history, the choice between freedom and responsibility was too often explained as dichotomous. What is needed is connective tissue between the two—a way of illustrating how the poles of each dichotomy are connected and can be employed in tandem.

Current research and theorizing suggests two such pieces of connective tissue: the concept of empathy, which has both a rational and an emotional quality, and the notion of proto-norms, which help to guide empathetic moral thinking along a professionally responsible path. First, then, empathy and its professional uses.

Research on empathy has employed somewhat different definitions of the term. All of them acknowledge a debt to feminist ethics, and within that the ethics of care. In Gilligan's original conceptualization (1982), care arises as a first response to human distress. It is then supplemented by self-sacrifice, followed by the realization that all involved in the particular moral problem are moral agents worthy of equal consideration and dignity (as opposed to self-sacrifice). Gilligan framed this growth in moral thinking as the "responsibility for the consequences of choice." She noted that the essence of moral decision is the exercise of choice and the willingness to take responsibility for that choice ... The criterion for judgment thus shifts from goodness to truth when the morality of action is assessed not on the basis of its appearance in the eyes of others, but in terms of the realities of its intention and consequence. (Gilligan, 1982, p. 150)

There is a human truth that emerges from care, Gilligan noted, and it is a universal truth of the caring moral self. Choice (freedom) and responsibility are connected through care (of self, of others, potentially of a professional role).

To care for others in this way requires empathy, what some (Slote, 2010) believe Hume actually meant when he used the word "sympathy" in his work. Disentangling empathy from sympathy can be difficult. "Empathy involves having the feelings of another (involuntarily) aroused in ourselves, as when we see another person in pain" (Slote, 2010, p. 15). An absence of empathy is sometimes easier to spot (Lifton, 1986) than the more subtle forms of the quality at work. Some philosophers have characterized adult empathy as "mindreading" (Prinz, 2007), but this characterization ignores substantial psychological and physiological evidence. Hoffman (2001) argues that individual empathy develops through several stages and that it is connected with prosocial, altruistic, and moral motivations. Infants can respond to the cries of others with "empathetic distress". In the cognitively mature person, however, "empathy isn't a total merging with or melting into the other; genuine and mature empathy doesn't deprive the empathic individual of her sense of being a different person from the person she empathizes with" (Sloate, 2010, p. 17). This construction of empathy differs significantly from that of Noddings (1984); Hoffman and Slote particularly connect empathy with moral agency because empathy is strongly connected with human action. The foregoing connection of empathy and action is crucial. An empathetic adult can understand and feel as another does without granting moral sanction. It is what writers do when they create villains who are "true to life," what biographers of leaders such as Hitler must do to truly understand their subjects, and it is what high levels of moral thinking demand. Ettema and Glasser, in their examination of investigative journalists (1998), reveal a form of professionally based empathy at work. These journalists are willing to suspend moral judgment in how they go about their work, even as they expose wrong doing and with it, a professional moral judgment rendered through facts and evidence. Here, the journalists care about their professional role, about the impact of that role on the public, and about a professional value that relies on "the facts speaking for themselves". As Slote notes, "I believe that empathy and the notion of empathetic caring for or about others in fact offer us a plausible criterion of moral evaluation" (2010, p. 21).

However, empathy can be only a starting place. Empathy still must have a moral standard, particularly for professionals who, in addition to the general morality, must also respond to the demands of a professional role. It allows individual actors to navigate between the two sets of standards. "This notion of commitment is argued to contribute to bounded decision making, to ease the problem of juggling multiple goals and co-ordinate group problem solving" (Gratch and Marsella, 2007).

Theoretically, the concept of proto-norms can provide that professional standard. As articulated by Christians (2010), the universal proto-norms of truthfulness, sacredness of life, and human dignity provide a normative standard that allows those who feel empathy for others to feel that empathy yet maintain the self-awareness to engage in moral evaluation. Proto-norms are the irreducible assumptions of moral thinking. Rather than being employed as individual "thought" elements, the proto-norms form a conceptual heuristic, a whole that is greater than the sum of the individual parts. As Christians notes, the concept of proto-norms demands that "the empirical remains embedded in human experience" rather than being abstracted from it. The proto-norms represent a set of basic beliefs about what it means to be human. For Christians, they forge the link between the "I" and the "thou" that so confounded Enlightenment meta-ethics (Christians, 2010). Furthermore, the proto-norms have an emotional as well as a cognitive component— proto-norms are not merely rational or merely emotional—they include elements of both. Thus, they reflect the contemporary understandings of neuroscience. The proto-norms in a single concept include that "firm handshake with the emotions" that effective ethical decision making demands. For journalists, who have loyalties to community, to the organizations for which they work, and to themselves as well as to more abstract ideals such as truth, employing the proto-norms—which is done intuitively as well as consciously—is what allows for nuanced ethical decision making under a variety of constraints. Journalistic actions that employ empathy for others while acting on the basis which does not violate, and sometimes foregrounds, the proto-norms can fuel the moral imagination and provide a way of analyzing the intellectual and emotional commitment that funds exceptional professional work. The proto-norms provide a normative boundary for human rationality. By basing journalistic work in the proto-norms of truthfulness, dignity and non-violence, and employing those standards informed by empathy, it is possible to see where journalisms' moral sentiments can honor both the freedom to act and accept the responsibility of doing so as a central component of ethical professional work. What follows is an example of that approach through viewing a film and subsequent interviews with both its creator and producer.

Enemies of the People: One Journalist's Vision of Truth and Reconciliation

Cambodian journalist Thet Sambath's (Lemkin and Sambath, 2009) father and brother were among the two million people believed to have been killed in the mid-1970s in the killing fields of Cambodia. For reasons both intensely personal and professional, Sambath set out to report the story of how the decisions about the killing field were made by individuals. Most of the people involved in the policy—from those who developed it to those who literally executed it—had never been charged with any crime. Many had never spoken publicly, even though their neighbors may have known about and even witnessed their crimes. Among them was Brother No. 2, Pol Pot's second in command, who still lives in Cambodia.

The documentary film, which was nominated for the Oscar for best documentary film in 2010, took Sambath most of a decade to shoot and report. First, Sambath focused his journalistic efforts on gaining the trust of Brother No. 2 and then getting him to speak about how the policy of the killing fields was developed. Gaining Brother No. 2's trust took three years, years in which Sambath visited him regularly and during which Brother No. 2 never spoke a word. Later, as trust between the two men did emerge, Brother No. 2 began to talk about his view of Cambodia during the 1970s and the rule of the Khmer Rouge. Although Brother No. 2 never executed anyone under the policy, ultimately and on camera he claimed credit for its development. Among his more chilling claims, that during this era of Cambodian history, Brother No. 2 trusted the party and the ideology it represented over and above the "people". In Brother No. 2's view, the implementation of a radical communist ideology was much more important than individual human life, in this case millions of human lives.

Sambath's repeated interviews with Brother No. 2 were superficially unemotional encounters. His initial questions were circumspect and almost tangential to the core of the story he was reporting. Yet, Sambath was careful never to let Brother No. 2 know that he had lost family members in the killing fields for fear of losing the trust of Brother No. 2 and hence bringing his reporting to an early end. However, his own lack of truthfulness concerned Sambath—by the end of the process, a decade after his first encounter—Sambath told Brother No. 2 about his personal loss. By then, Brother No. 2 was in the process of being charged with war crimes, but he accepted Sambath's statements without recanting what he had said earlier. In some sense, he appeared to regard Sambath as a friend, although it was a peculiar friendship by any measure.

Sambath's reporting did not stop there. He knew that others had carried out the orders from the central government, and he set out to interview those Cambodians as well. In perhaps the most chilling scene in the film, one of the Cambodians who was directly and personally involved in the killing demonstrated for Sambath how he sliced the throats of his countrymen, shifting his grip on his knife and changing the way he cut into human flesh when his hand became tired. These killers admitted what they did on camera. Sambath also questioned others who lived in the village and knew of the crimes and those who committed them. These Cambodians said that there were fields where they refused to drink because they believed them polluted by human corpses, that they knew that those who had committed these atrocities still lived in the villages, and they were afraid to behave differently toward them because they remembered this horrific time in Cambodian history.

Sambath's years of effort in the form of a trunk full of video tape he kept at his home was ultimately joined by a Western filmmaker Rob Lemkin who helped Sambath edit his store of information into a documentary film. In interviews, both men said that they had pursued this story because it represented a journalistic truth that needed to be told, primarily for the Cambodian people but secondarily for the rest of the world.

That Sambath is a journalistic hero there is little doubt. But there is equally little doubt that it was emotion that founded his drive to get the story and report it thoroughly. Although Sambath never used the Western concept when he talked about how he was able to get people to admit what they had done on camera, it was evident that he empathized with them by understanding their motives (ideology and/or "following orders") while sustaining his own moral judgment. The drive to get the story, of course, is the journalistic drive for truth, but it is a truth that is emotionally connected to a commitment to the sacredness of life and to human dignity—both to the Cambodians who were killed during this genocide and to their killers. Sambath also negotiated between freedom and responsibility; he exercised his moral agency by even attempting to "get" this particular story, yet he felt responsible not just for its content but how it was reported. Sambath's efforts can be thought of as a professional attempt at truth and reconciliation—a truth that acknowledges a genocidal past, human culpability in it, and provides an alternate vision to audiences through the actions of a single human being. Even the most casual viewer of the film comes away with an understanding of the moral sentiments that propelled it. Far from overwhelming rationality, it is the sentiments that seem to sustain clear thinking in times of stress. Sambath's efforts also focus on the importance of rationality coupled with emotion. In fact, it was not until another journalist helped Sambath edit his tapes—a somewhat more detached and professionally-oriented effort than the struggle to get the story itself on tape—that the film itself emerged. While the Western editor was hardly unmoved by the piece, he also brought some professional skills to the project that Sambath, for complex reasons, was unable to exercise. Their partnership illustrates the relationship between the emotions based in the ethical proto-norms and the rationality needed to exercise that understanding in a professional context. Interviews and comments from the two men about the film itself make this level of professional partnership clear.

This example, of course, provides both an illustration and leads to questions. The first is a question that philosophers have been stumbling on since the Enlightenment: how is it that people, acting as individuals as well as in a professional capacity—can chip away at this ethical bedrock? If we intuitively understand the proto-norms, why are we so capable of ignoring them? How is it that the proto-norms can provide some insight into work such as Sambath's as well as the actions of the radio journalists in Rwanda who encouraged their listeners to commit genocide? The foregoing question speaks to individual responsibility, yet journalists today largely work in organizations. How might it be possible to make news organizations collectively responsible—to develop organizations more capable of sustaining the insights of the proto-norms for their individual employees—is another question that extends this discussion. These are questions this essay will not address, but readers should not be unmindful of them.

However, coupling emotion with logic provides a compelling heuristic with which to understand how journalists navigate between the professional ideals of freedom and responsibility. Far from being dichotomous, these ideals should be viewed as connected to each other—the professional "I" and "thou" which make sense only when considered in tandem. The film *Enemies of the People*, and its development and creation, provide powerful evidence that responsibility and freedom appropriately connected produce the sort of professional, moral exemplar that journalists of many cultures can aspire to.

REFERENCES

ARISTOTLE (1999) "Nichomachean Ethics".

AUDI, ROBERT (2005) *The Good in the Right: a theory of intuition and intrinsic value*, Princeton, NJ: Princeton University Press.

BUSEMEYER, JEROME R., DIMPERIO, ERIC and JESSUP, RYAN K. (2007) "Integrating Emotional Processes into Decision-making Models", in: Wayne D. Gray (Ed.), *Integrated models of cognitive systems*, Oxford: Oxford University Press.

CHRISTIANS, CLIFFORD G. (2010) "Response: theories of morality in three dimensions", in: R. Fortner and M. Fackler (Eds), *Ethics & Evil in the Public Sphere: media, universal values and global development*, Cresskill, NJ: Hampton Press, pp. 335–46.

CHRISTIANS, CLIFFORD G, FERRE, J. P. and FACKLER, M. (1993) *Good News: social ethics and the press*, New York: Oxford University Press.

COLEMAN, RENITA and WILKINS, LEE (2002) "Searching for the Ethical Journalist: an exploratory study of the ethical development of news workers", *Journal of Mass Media Ethics* 17(3), pp. 209–55.

COLEMAN, RENITA and WILKINS, LEE (2004) "The Moral Development of Journalists: a comparison with other professions and a model for predicting high quality ethical reasoning", *Journalism & Mass Communication Quarterly* 81(3), pp. 511–27.

D'ARMS, JUSTIN and JACOBSON, DANIEL (2000) "Sentiment and Value", *Ethics* 110, pp. 722–48.

DE WAAL, and FRANS, B. M. (1996) *Good Natured: the origins of right and wrong in humans and other animals*, Cambridge, MA: Harvard University Press.

ETTEMA, JAMES S. and GLASSER, THEODORE L. (1998) *Custodians of Conscience*, New York: Columbia University Press.

GAZZANIGA, MICHAEL S. (2005) *The Ethical Brain: the science of our moral dilemmas*, New York: HarperCollins.

GILLIGAN, CAROL (1982) *In a Different Voice: psychological theory and women's development*, Cambridge, MA: Harvard University Press.

GRATCH, JONATHAN and MARSELLA, STACY (2007) "The Architectural Role of Emotion in Cognitive Systems", in: W. D. Gray (Ed.), *Integrated models of cognition systems*, Oxford: Oxford University Press.

HAUSER, MARC D. (2006) *Moral Minds: how nature designed our universal sense of right and wrong*, New York: HarperCollins.

HOFFMAN, MARTIN (2001) *Empathy and Moral Development: implications for care and justice*, Cambridge: Cambridge University Press.

HUME, DAVID (1977 [1739]) *A Treatise of Human Nature*, Oxford: Oxford University Press.

KOHLBERG, LAURENCE (1981) *Essays on Moral Development,* Vol. 1, *The philosophy of moral development*, New York: Harper & Row.

KOHLBERG, LAURENCE (1984) *The Psychology of Moral Development: the nature and validity of moral stages*, San Francisco: Harper & Row.

LEMKIN, ROB and SAMBATH, THET (2009) *Enemies of the People,* Documentary Film, viewed February 2010, Columbia: MO.

LIFTON, ROBERT J. (1986) *The Nazi Doctors: medical killing and the psychology of genocide*, New York: Basic Books.

MERRILL, JOHN (1974) *The Imperative of Freedom: a philosophy of public communication*, New York: Hastings House Book.

MILL, JOHN STUART (1859) "On Liberty".

MOSER, PAUL K. (1990) *Rationality in Action: contemporary approaches*, Cambridge: Cambridge University Press.

NICHOLS, SHAUN (2004) *Sentimental Rules: on the natural foundation of moral judgment*, Oxford: Oxford University Press.

NODDINGS, NEL (1984) *Caring: a feminine approach to ethics and moral education*, Berkeley: University of California Press.

PIAGET, JEAN (1965) *The Moral Judgment of the Child*, New York: The Free Press.

PRINZ, JESSE J. (2007) *The Emotional Construction of Morals*, Oxford: Oxford University Press.

RAO, SHAKUNTALA and LEE, SEOW TING (2005) "Globalizing Media Ethics: an assessment of universal ethics among international political journalists", *Journal of Mass Media Ethics* 20(2/3), pp. 99–120.

REST, JAMES R. (1986) *Moral Development: advances in research and theory*, New York: Praeger.

REST, JAMES R., NARVAEZ, DARCIA, BEBEAU, MURIEL J. and THOMA, STEPHAN J. (1999) *Postconventional Moral Thinking: a neo-Kohlbergian approach*, Mahwah, NJ: Lawrence Erlbaum Associates.

SLOTE, MICHAEL (2010) *Moral Sentimentalism*, Oxford: Oxford University Press.

SMITH, ADAM (2010 [1759]) *Theory of Moral Sentiments*, New York: Cosimo Classics.

WARD, STEPHEN J. A. (2004) *The Invention of Journalism Ethics*, Montreal and Kingston: McGill University Press.

WILKINS, LEE and COLEMAN, RENITA (2005) *The Moral Media: how journalists reason about ethics*, Mahwah, NJ: Lawrence Erlbaum & Associates.

WRIGHT, ROBERT (1994) *The Moral Animal: why we are the way we are: the new science of evolutionary psychology*, New York: Vintage Books.

NEGOTIATING GLOBAL AND LOCAL JOURNALISM ETHICS
A case-study of how a local Dubai radio talk show covered the arrest of a couple for kissing in public

James Piecowye

Nightline *is an English-language talk radio format program broadcast in Dubai, United Arab Emirates, on 103.8 FM. As the host of* Nightline*, I try to balance local sensibility, regulations, institutional codes of conduct, regional morality, and global media ethics. Through investigations and interviews,* Nightline *regularly pushes the boundaries of what is defined as acceptable programming in the United Arab Emirates. In this paper, I discuss one particular case-study which highlights the difficulty of negotiating global and local journalism ethics in a predominantly Arab-Muslim region.*

Introduction

The application of studies in ethics to the world of radio broadcasting is complicated, contradictory and, at times, difficult to comprehend from within global media studies. Gordon et al. (1996) point out the difficulty of applying philosophical and ethical principles to journalism in the real world. The application of ethics is complicated and problematic because of the ambiguity of philosophical principles, the tenacity of local laws, and the largely misunderstood enculturation process that informs the actions and thoughts of individuals. Thus, it has come to be believed by many that ethical decision making, in a practical context, is complicated because it is overly influenced by environmental, cultural, and other inherent restrictions. This case-study addresses how a culturally sensitive issue was handled on a live radio show called *Nightline*, aired on a Dubai-based English-language radio station, Dubai Eye 103.8 FM. In this case-study I will examine the content of the program in which we discussed the arrest of a British couple who were found kissing in public. My goal in this paper is to show how local cultural codes of conduct and legal regulations bear heavily on ethical decision making among foreign-language radio broadcasters in the United Arab Emirates (UAE). I argue that while there is increasing hybridization of culture and media practices, major ethical decisions continue to be influenced less by Western theories of press freedom and responsibilities and more by local ethics codes, laws, and a fear of punishment.

Radio in the UAE

Dubai Eye 103.8 FM is the UAE's only all-talk English-language format radio station broadcasting 24 hours a day. Dubai Eye is broadcast terrestrially and streamed over the Internet. Dubai Eye is one of several stations owned and operated by the Arabian Radio Network (ARN), a subsidiary of the Arab Media Group (AMG) which is owned by Dubai Holding, a Dubai government entity (Arabian Radio Network, 2009). While Dubai Eye is a local UAE broadcast operation, the management of the radio station is entirely made up of Western expatriates. For example, the Chief Operating Officer of ARN is an Australian expatriate, Steve Smith. The programming director of Dubai Eye is Susan Perry, a British expatriate with several years of broadcasting experience in the United Kingdom. The producers and core group of show hosts are, collectively, from the United Kingdom, Australia, South Africa, New Zealand, Canada, and the Philippines.

Radio and, in particular, English-language Talk Radio, is a relatively new format in Dubai. Radio itself is new to the UAE compared to broadcast history in the West. Prior to 1964 there was no locally operated radio in the region; residents had to depend on programming originating from the British Representatives offices in what is now the Emirate of Sharjah (Zayed University College of Communication and Media Sciences, 1999). Radio broadcasting in the Arab world is relatively young with the first indigenous Arab broadcasting entity being formed when the Jordanian government acquired the transmitter in Ramallah previously used by the British government. As the colonial forces of Britain and France departed the Arab world it was not unusual for local governments to acquire radio facilities left behind and incorporate them as state institutions. Early Arab broadcasting faced many challenges including securing the rights to frequencies and finding personnel with the skill and experience to manage and deliver sustainable quality content (Zayed University College of Media and Communication Sciences, 1999). The first indigenous radio station in what is now the UAE was established in Sharjah in 1964. In 1969 the Abu Dhabi government also established a radio station that was programmed almost exclusively with Arabic-language content. Abu Dhabi Radio was renamed United Arab Emirates Radio in 1971. From 1971 to today several private or quasi-private terrestrial broadcast radio stations have been formed in Dubai, Abu Dhabi, Sharjah, Ajman and Fujairah (Zayed University College of Media and Communication Sciences, 1999).

The newest radio network in the nation is the ARN which was founded in September 2001 and joined the AMG in March 2005, consolidating television, radio and print interests. At the height of its success AMG was home to over 20 media brands including television, radio, print, digital, outdoor advertising, printing and event management. After a reorganization of the company in 2009, AMG became home to seven radio stations including Dubai Eye 103.8 FM, the English-language, multicultural talk radio station.

Nightline on Dubai Eye

The program *Nightline* is broadcast weekly from Sunday through Wednesday, 8 to 10 p.m. *Nightline* has a very basic format. During the show's first hour a question is posed to the listeners and they are asked to call in or SMS (instant messaging) their opinions. The second hour of *Nightline* offers an in-depth interview with studio guests. In this part of the program audience input is not generally solicited as the host interviews the guests for approximately 45 minutes in what is generally regarded as a coffeehouse-style conversation which is relaxed and informative. *Nightline* is produced by Alix Capper-Murdoch, a veteran to UAE Radio. I am the host of *Nightlight* and have been hosting the show for the past five years. I am a Canadian expatriate who has been living in Dubai for the past 11 years and also an associate professor in the College of Communication and Media Sciences at Zayed University's Dubai campus. The selection of guests and topics on *Nightline*, over the years, has been very broad: ministers, scholars, academics, university professors, community activists, and local and international newsmakers have all been guests on the show.

Nightline's success in the region can be attributed to its ability to connect with an English-speaking audience. In order to engage listeners, *Nightline* actively uses new technologies such as SMS, Twitter, Facebook, Livestream, podomatic, and blogs. While no independent audience statistics are available, ARN management claims that its own in-house research shows that Dubai Eye has 110,000 listeners at any given time with the average listener staying tuned in for more than one hour. A cursory examination might lead an observer to suggest that ARN and Dubai Eye, with programs such as *Nightline*, are not really different from other global broadcast organizations; the differences, however, can be found in the rules and codes that govern content.

Media Law and Journalistic Codes of Ethics in the UAE

The UAE has an interesting broadcast environment because of the country's relatively new and flourishing broadcast industries. The UAE was established as a sovereign federation in 1971 and its first media laws were only formalized in the 1980s. Currently, new media laws are in the works and the older ones are being revised but they have yet to be implemented, creating an ambiguous situation for those working in the industry. A concept such as press freedom, which can easily become contentious, is still under negotiation. While there have been mixed reviews of the impending legal structures of the UAE draft Media Activities Law, uncertainty among journalists about the new law's legal provisions concerning freedom and independence has prompted many media practitioners to exercise guarded optimism.

While the current 30-year-old Press and Publications Law and the draft Media Activities Law apply principally to print media, broadcasting continues to be regulated by local government and Free Media Zone standards. Recently, the UAE National Media Council (NMC), which oversees media regulation in the country, has launched a joint drive with the Telecommunications Regulatory Authority (TRA) to make regulations transparent for the audio-visual industry. According to a draft document, while TRA would handle technical issues relating to spectrum allocation and equipment licensing, NMC would take care of content regulation. When applied to the UAE landscape, the new rules would serve as a centralized regulatory umbrella covering federal and local broadcasting operations in addition to those based in Free Media Zones.

In 2007 the UAE Journalist Association agreed on a code of ethics for its members. This code of ethics consists of 26 clauses that are not legally but morally binding for its members. Two of the clauses are significant to mention here as they relate to the case-study to be discussed later. The first clause states, "Journalists should not seek to provoke or inflame public feelings by any means or use means of excitement and deception or dishonest reporting." The second clause reminds broadcasters and journalists that,

"Islam is a basic and important component of UAE culture, values and traditions, and the respect of divine religions and traditions and values of nations takes centre stage at the mandatory code of ethics of the media and should not be offended or desecrated by any forms." Both of these clauses serve as guidelines and reminders to journalists and broadcasters, especially Western expatriates, that the UAE has a different media environment, in content and style, when compared to the West. Other regional broadcast organizations like Abu Dhabi Media Company, Dubai Media Incorporated and Sharjah Media Incorporated as well as UAE-based Free Media Zones like Dubai Media City and Abu Dhabi Two-Four54 Media Zone have also evolved their own codes of ethics.

Dubai Eye's programming policy also attempts to set guidelines on what can and cannot be broadcast. The Dubai Eye internal broadcast policy document suggests:

> There are an infinite number of comments which should not be broadcast on *Dubai Eye*. The rule of thumb is to check with the Head of Programming in advance of discussing any subject listed, and, at all times, to use common sense and consider the response of our friends in the government and our listeners when we frame any question or comment. There are very few subjects that are off limits—the main point is that they are dealt with in a manner which is non-offensive. (Arabian Radio Network, 2009)

There is no room for criticism of the State in radio broadcasting in the UAE. It is clearly written that, "No presenter has a right to question the judicial system, to question the decisions and policies of the Dubai Government, any federal ministry, or the leadership of the country." Topics related to sex can also be highly problematic as the policy states, "Sex, subjectively should not be discussed. For many of our listeners, it is seen as an offensive subject. Homosexuality is illegal, and as such, should not be discussed on air" states the policy. Also clearly stated is, "Criticism of the royal family will not be tolerated on air, nor will any effort to undermine any individual member of the surrounding Gulf States." The overriding direction from the corporation, when it comes to broadcasting content, as stated in the programming policy is, "the main point is that [topics] are dealt with in a way which is non-offensive. This is why you have been selected to present on *Dubai Eye*, why you have been given the privilege to broadcast live across Dubai, because you are able to retain this balance on air whilst mediating the discussion" (Arabian Radio Network, 2009).

Journalists and media professionals find themselves in a precarious situation as they operate under the legal guidance of antiquated laws and a series of non-legal binding codes of ethics that attempt to bring clarity and guidance to content creation. When discussions of journalism ethics, most often influenced by Western scholarship, is added to the equation, the situation is further complicated.

Negotiating Global and Local Media Ethics

Christians (2008) points out that the mass media today are in a constant state of negotiation and nowhere is this more apparent than in the UAE. It is difficult not to agree with Christians when he writes that ethical decision making might be best described as a world of ideas. But the issue that we constantly return to as we interact with "this world of ideas," in an academic sense, is how do we relate the larger philosophical, and more abstract, ideas to the media reality we live in? The hope, as Christians suggests, is that through the use of ethical analysis, standardized language, and common systematized approaches we will gain some consistency in how we understand and address ethical issues and concerns in the professional world. The question we return to and one we stated in the introduction of this paper is: how can we navigate between the academic/ hypothetical and the real world of ethical decision making in media and journalism practices in the UAE?

It is my belief that what links theory to practice in journalism ethics is culture (as suggested in the articles of Ayish and Ward in this issue of the journal: Ayish, 2011; Ward, 2011). It can easily be argued that all culture today is a hybrid of the global and local to some degree and this hybridization of culture is at the core of ethics and broadcast journalism practices in the UAE. In order to consider culture and how we have come to see it as hybrid it is necessary to understand the term culture itself. Williams (1981) suggests that culture might be best understood as the general process of intellectual, spiritual, and aesthetic development of a society. Using this definition we can explain not only what culture is, in the broader sense of the term, but we can also begin to understand how cultures can come to be understood in a hybrid sense. It is possible, as Canclini (1993) suggests, to think of hybrid culture as not having a coherence or static body of specific signifiers but to be in a constant state of change and development; that is "permanent transformation" based on what is going on in the environment. It is the environmental juxtaposition between what is happening in the UAE and what is imported to the UAE, both physically and psychologically, that becomes problematic when applied to the media environment.

Culture is an often ignored issue in the negotiation of journalism ethics because it is considered to be fluid in its composition; but culture is of paramount importance. The problem of the fluidity of culture is that because it is simultaneously hidden and ever-present we tend to marginalize the influence of culture on the creation and dissemination of media products. Bennett describes the issue aptly:

> popular culture is definable neither as the culture of the people, produced by and for themselves, nor as an administered culture produced for them. Rather, it consists of those cultural forms and practices—varying in content from one historical period to another—which constitute the terrain on which dominant, subordinate and oppositional cultural values and ideologies meet and intermingle, in different mixes and permutations, vying with one another in their attempts to secure the spaces within which they can become influential in framing and organizing popular experience and consciousness. (1986, pp. 18–19)

The hybridity of culture Bennett alludes to in the above quote can be understood as a fundamental building block of everything we do. We are influenced by culture as much as we are part of culture which creates a precarious situation in cultural industries and in this particular case radio broadcasting in the UAE. The precarious situation arises because of the confluence of Western and Middle Eastern ideas and expectations of the role of media. As we move around the globe we interact with different cultural environments that are informing different audiences creating a hybrid culture. Hybridization, of course, is not an issue if those people creating media content and those people consuming media content are products of the same cultural environment but today this is highly unlikely given the ease with which people and ideas are spread globally. What is happening is the cultural underpinnings of local media are blurred as expatriate content creators migrate elsewhere in search of better opportunities. These content creators have to deal with the issues of local culture, hybridity, and the way in which they themselves navigate differences. Take a Canadian broadcaster operating in the UAE like myself. We are confronted with understanding Islamic values and restrictions of freedom of expression. These two issues would never have been part of Canadian culture and journalism practice and require a fundamental realignment of one's thinking. An argument can be made that you cannot simply rethink your cultural foundations. Here we are left in an interesting situation; we have the cultural underpinnings of the UAE that dictate how the media will operate, we have the varied expectations of consumers with their own particular cultural experiences, and we have the content creators themselves coming from another, entirely different, cultural perspective, all intermingling to create and define a dynamic media environment.

Case-study of the Arrest and Conviction of the British Couple for Kissing in Public: Practicalities of Broadcast Journalism in the UAE

Considering the legal rules governing media in the UAE, the code of ethics of the Journalist Association, Islamic morality and various institutional regulations regarding programming in the UAE, it is surprising that a program like *Nightline* even exists. However, there has been no dearth of topics one can talk about on *Nightline*, given the way the UAE constantly vacillates between trying to project an image of itself, on one hand as a conservative Muslim state adhering to the strict principles of Islam and, on the other hand, a more liberal Muslim state with global ambitions especially in the financial sector. It is this push and pull in public sensibility that makes programs like *Nightline* engaging.

At times the UAE seems to be caught between the global and local, alternately wanting the benefits of a Westernized laissez faire economy with all the claims that come with such economic development and, at the same time, strengthening its more conservative Islamic cultural roots. Over the years, on *Nightline*, we have discussed wide-ranging topics which clearly point to the global–local negotiation that is taking place in the Arab world and more specifically in the UAE. Topics of conversations on the show have included the whimsical such as breaking Guinness world records to the more serious such as spouse abuse. Programming on *Nightline* has been aided by the fact that Dubai, in particular, and the UAE, in general, have become not only a tourist destination but also home to many diverse cultures that have competing views on what is acceptable and unacceptable behavior and morality. *Nightline* plays to these competing views, simultaneously championing local cultural sensibilities but also introducing global ways of thinking about issues and addressing them in a public forum. The complications in navigating the local and the global begin with the broadcast media facilities owned and regulated by UAE citizens but overwhelmingly staffed by expatriates. This creates challenges in the decisions of what should and should not be discussed over public airwaves. Case in point is the increasing number of Western tourists finding themselves on the wrong side of the law for drinking in public and for public displays of affection.

Between December 2009 and August 2010 there seemed to be a spike in the number of Westerners who were being arrested, prosecuted, and convicted for offending Islam, in particular the number of people being arrested for public displays of affection between men and women. An incident that grabbed media attention took place in November 2009. In this case, a British expatriate, living in Dubai, and a British tourist were accused of committing a sexual act, kissing, in the upscale neighborhood of Jumeirah Beach in Dubai. Ayman Najafi and Charlotte Adams, both in their twenties, were arrested after an Emirati woman claimed they exchanged a passionate kiss in a restaurant where she and her daughter were having dinner. The couple was convicted in January 2010 and sentenced to one month in jail, to pay a fine of 1000 dirhams (about $270) and each were to be deported after serving their sentences. The UAE adheres to strict Islamic rules and bans sex outside of marriage and kissing has been categorized as a "sex act".

On *Nightline* we decided to do a call-in program about the topic of how expatriate communities navigate between the Western and Islamic cultures of the UAE. Given the timing of the program and the media coverage of the Najafi and Adams case, we were pretty certain that there would be some negative reactions expressed on the program but chose to go ahead with the show. The conversation was initiated by asking listeners how well they thought Western and UAE morality and culture coexisted in Dubai. The Najafi and Adams case was mentioned but not discussed in detail. In the course of the conversation listeners were also asked how expatriates and Emiratis might go about balancing different cultural perspectives given that Dubai has become a hybrid cultural space. I gave examples of the existence of malls, hotels, restaurants, and bars but also how education, sports, and marital expectations were also influenced by cultural hybridization. When the phone-lines were opened we took three calls. Below is an edited transcript of caller responses.

Caller 1:
Hi! I only have a couple of points that I want to make. The reason why I find this situation a little bit infuriating here in Dubai is because you got one rule for celebrities and another entirely different rules for the locals . . . For instance, when Angelina Jolie came here with her six kids and her boyfriend and everyone knew about it the police did nothing. And I also recall Lindsay Lohan when she came here with her lesbian lover, stayed at the hotel, was a very public event. So, I take issue of the fact that they got one rule for the people who bring commercial values to Dubai and an entirely different rule for those living here . . . It's got to be consistent. The other problem that I have is when a local or someone who is religious makes an accusation on somebody else, basically their word is against yours. And unfortunately when a situation like that comes up, the police are more likely to believe those who are conservative because they went through the trouble of making a complaint.

Caller 2:
My point is when Dubai markets itself internationally it doesn't market itself as an Islamic country with Islamic beliefs. If you look at the Emirates airline brochures and advertisements that are filled with people with swimsuits on beaches and are having romantic dinners and roaming around with their kids . . . If they want us to respect local values and cultures, that's fine. But I think they got to stop sending mixed messages. If this is an Islamic country and they want us to abide by Islamic rules, which I have no problem with, they've got to really telegraph that clearly to the world. But that's what comes with the conflict that they want the tourism dollar. If, for example, you were booking a holiday to Iran, if I can use that as an example, you would be very much aware that you have to have your Abhaya [veil] that is a very strict code of conduct. You come to Dubai and lines are not so definite. For example, men walking hand in hand in Dubai is a cultural thing which is accepted, that would not be accepted in many similar Western

countries. Whereas, a lady walking in a covered manner is accepted, but if a peck on the cheek is too much or not too much, for some it is, for some it isn't but the government I think are responsible and are not laying the line more clearly.

Caller 3:
The government has a responsibility to be clear because they market Dubai as a hedonistic shopping paradise with five-star hotels, with everything laid on including alcohol. So when all goes wrong they say what happened here but in reality they can say we're Muslim country, that's fine, but telegraph it more clearly to the people who are spending their hard-earned annual holiday here and bringing their money to the country.

In the examples from the calls to *Nightline* transcribed above, the three callers were openly speaking about issues which, according to Islam, are deemed as inappropriate and illegal. Caller 1 talked about "boyfriends" and "lesbianism," practices which may exist in the UAE, but are definitely not spoken in a public context. The UAE Journalist Association, in an attempt to clarify for its members how content should be formulated to meet the challenges, has suggested that first and foremost "Journalists should not seek to provoke or inflame public feelings by any means or use means of excitement and deception or dishonest reporting." By speaking about a situation where a couple is prosecuted and convicted for an illegal sex act, it is possible that *Nightline* was breaking the code of ethics of journalists and this could have led to professional and possibly legal repercussions. Further, the UAE Journalist Association is also very clear that it expects its members to respect Islam. By the callers talking about dating and homosexuality as well as pointing fingers at celebrities being exempt from Islamic laws it is very possible that someone could have interpreted the content of the show as being critical of the government. Both of the above-stated clauses serve as reminders to journalists and broadcasters, especially Western expatriates, that the UAE is indeed a different media environment and that they need to be vigilant about how they present ideas or challenge local sensibilities.

The management of Dubai Eye stresses that there are few subjects that are off limits. Yet, there is no room for criticism of the state; no broadcaster has a right to question the judicial system, to question the decisions and policies of the Dubai Government, any federal ministry, or the leadership of the country. Sex cannot be discussed and since homosexuality is illegal, it cannot be mentioned on air (unpublished Programming Guide). Again red flags went up when callers, such as caller 2, suggested that the state is at fault when it came to an incident like Najafi and Adams because of the mixed messages being sent to the public (i.e., contradictory assertions that we have an Islamic state but have advertisements which display open alcohol consumption). Such calls could have been misconstrued as being critical of the state, critical of the judiciary and the police. What this type of conversation points to is the cultural changes taking place in the UAE because of ongoing hybridization, foreign influences given the large expatriate population, and ease of obtaining Western media content. Contradictions emerge, however, when the UAE attempts to lure tourists by presenting itself as an open and progressive society and simultaneously attempts to maintain a more conservative and Islamic cultural base.

As a broadcaster I need to constantly be on guard concerning how I interact with callers. I cannot be seen as taking sides with callers who express ideas which might be perceived as anti-government. For my part of the conversation I do not add any comments or editorialize when the callers are speaking; I attempt to sound neutral about the topic. In this case, there was, however, general uneasiness in the studio because of the prospect that listeners to the show might understand the conversation as a form of criticism of the UAE government and initiate a complaint or that the management of the station themselves might deem the conversation as a veiled criticism of the state and outright cancel the show.

Conclusion

Being a broadcaster in the UAE is a challenge because cultural rules play a role in deciding media content. On *Nightline* there is a constant push and pull between what content might be acceptable and unacceptable. There is always concern not only about what is being broadcast as being arbitrarily interpreted as violating Islamic laws but also about the diversity of the audiences and their reactions to the content. The UAE is a potpourri of different cultures because of the high number of immigrants from South Asia, Philippines, Egypt, and Africa who live and work in the UAE, many of whom listen to English radio. Different cultures bring to the content different interpretations based on their own history. As a broadcaster, discussing controversial topics such as the arrest and conviction of the British couple for kissing in public, one always has to consider if the discussion would violate or hurt local religious and cultural sentiments or the sentiments of some listeners. As a host of the show, I have to keep in mind Dubai Eye's own programming policy, UAE Journalist Association codes, and the laws of the country. As the station rules suggest, there is no room for criticism of the state in radio broadcasting in the UAE. While this directive is problematic because many of the issues that are discussed in the call-in segment of the show could easily be interpreted in some form to be questioning the actions of the state, I have to constantly skirt around the issues to avoid any direct criticism of the government or the Royal family.

It has been argued in this paper that decisions about content in UAE radio broadcasting and on shows, such as *Nightline*, are made with little focus on press freedom and more out of fear of the state's action against content it might deem culturally inappropriate for broadcast. The fear of offending a listener who might call the police and set the criminal justice system into motion is always at the back of the minds of all broadcast journalists like me in the UAE. While the UAE is gradually becoming hybridized in media practices (many of the broadcasters are expatriates), content is still largely influenced by local Islamic cultural and ethics codes rather than codes and rules imported from the West.

REFERENCES

ARABIAN RADIO NETWORK (2009) *Dubai Eye 103.8, Mission, Vision and Programming Policy*, Dubai: Arabian Radio Network.

AYISH, MUHAMMAD (2011) "Television Reality Shows in the Arab World: the case for a 'glocalized' media ethics", *Journalism Studies* 12(6), pp. 768–79.

BENNETT, TONY (1986) "The Politics of the Popular and Popular Culture", in: Tony Bennett, Colin Mercer and Janet Wollacott (Eds), *Popular Culture and Social Relations*, Philadelphia: Open University Press, pp. 6–21.

CANCLINI, NESTOR GARCIA (1993) "The Hybrid: a conversation with Margarita Zires, Raymundo Mier, and Mabel Piccini", *Boundary* 20(3), pp. 11–42.

CHRISTIANS, CLIFFORD (2008) "Media Ethics in Education", *Journalism Communication Monographs* 9(4), pp. 181–221.

GORDON, DAVID, KITTROSS, JOHN and REUSS, CAROL (1996) *Controversies in Media Ethics*, White Plains, NY: Longman.

WARD, STEPHEN J. A. (2011) "Ethical Flourishing as Aim of Global Media Ethics", *Journalism Studies* 12(6), pp. 738–46.

WILLIAMS, RAYMOND (1981) *Culture*, London: Fontana.

ZAYED UNIVERSITY COLLEGE OF COMMUNICATION AND MEDIA SCIENCES (1999) *COM201*, Electronic Textbook, Dubai: Zayed University College of Communication and Media Sciences.

Index

INDEX

INDEX

INDEX

INDEX

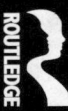

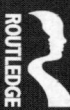

Related titles from Routledge

Foreign Correspondence

Edited by Maxwell John Hamilton and Regina G. Lawrence

Despite the importance of foreign news, its history, transformation and indeed its future have not been much studied. The need to redress this neglect and the desire to assess the impact of new media technologies on the future of journalism, including foreign correspondence, provide the motivation for this stimulating, exciting and thought-provoking book.

While the old economic models supporting news have crumbled in the wake of new media technologies, these changes have the potential to bring new and improved ways to inform people of foreign news. Journalism is being transformed by the effortlessly quick sharing of information across national boundaries. As such, we need to reconsider foreign correspondence and explore where such reporting is headed. This book discusses the current state and future prospects for foreign correspondence across the full range of media platforms, and assesses developments in the reporting of overseas news for audiences, governments and foreign policy in both contemporary and historical settings around the globe.

This book was originally published as a special issue of *Journalism Studies*.

May 2012: 246 x174: 160 pp
Hb: 978-0-415-62289-9
£85 / $135

JOURNALISM PRACTICE

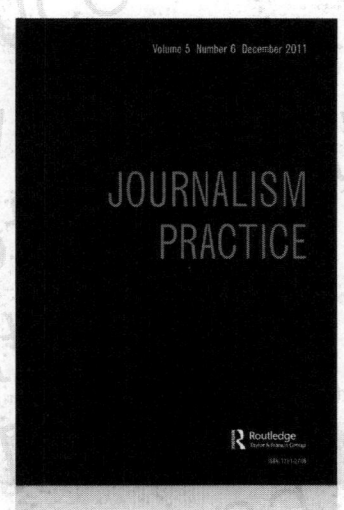

Volume 5 Number 6 December 2011

Editor: **Bob Franklin**, *Cardiff University, UK*

Journalism Practice provides opportunities for reflective, critical and research-based studies focused on the professional practice of journalism. *Journalism Practice*'s primary concern is to analyse and explore issues of practice and professional relevance. The journal aims to complement current trends to expansion in the teaching and analysis of journalism practice within the academy, reflection on the emergence of a reflective curriculum and thereby help to consolidate journalism as an intellectual discipline within the landscape of higher education.

Journalism Practice is devoted to: the study and analysis of significant issues arising from journalism as a field of professional practice; relevant developments in journalism training and education, as well as the construction of a reflective curriculum for journalism; analysis of journalism practice across the distinctive but converging media platforms of magazines, newspapers, online, radio and television; and the provision of a public space for practice-led, scholarly contributions from journalists as well as academics.

www.tandfonline.com/rjop

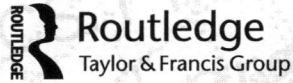

Routledge
Taylor & Francis Group

JOURNALISM STUDIES

LISTED IN THE THOMSON REUTERS
SOCIAL SCIENCES INDEX®

Editor: **Bob Franklin,** *Cardiff University, UK*

Journalism Studies is an international peer-reviewed journal, published by Routledge, Taylor & Francis, which provides a forum for the critical discussion and study of journalism as both a subject of academic inquiry and an arena of professional practice. The journal's editorial board and contributors reflect the intellectual interests of a global community of academics and practitioners concerned with addressing and analysing all aspects of journalism scholarship, journalism practice and journalism education.

Journalism Studies pursues an ambitious agenda which seeks to explore the widest possible range of media within which journalism is conducted (including multimedia), as well as analysing the full range of journalistic specialisms from sport and entertainment coverage to the central concerns of news, politics, current affairs, public relations and advertising.

www.tandfonline.com/rjos

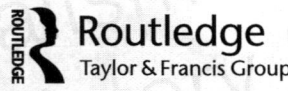
Routledge
Taylor & Francis Group